Dr. Gregory Ellis's
Ultimate Diet Secrets Lite

The 100% Weight Loss and Weight Control Solution
Featuring Dr. Ellis's 100/100 Plan

Gregory S. Ellis, PhD, CNS

First Edition

AN IMPORTANT CAUTION TO MY READERS

This book is not a medical manual and cannot take the place of personalized medical and nutritional advice from a qualified physician. Readers are urged to consult a physician or other health-care professional before beginning any diet.

The author and publisher cannot guarantee that the information and advice in this book are safe and proper for every reader. For that reason, this book is sold without warranties or guarantees of any kind, express or implied, and the author and publisher disclaim any liability, loss or damage caused by the contents.

If you do not wish to be bound by these cautions and conditions, you may return your copy to the publisher for a full refund.

Targeted Body Systems Publishing * Glen Mills, PA 19342

Dr. Gregory Ellis's
Ultimate Diet Secrets Lite

The 100% Weight Loss and Weight Control Solution
Featuring Dr. Ellis's 100/100 Plan

By Gregory S. Ellis, PhD, CNS

Published by:

Targeted Body Systems Publishing
68 Skyline Drive
Glen Mills, PA 19342
Orders @ www.ultimatedietsecrets.com
800-337-7041

Copyright © 2003 by Gregory S. Ellis

Except for brief quotations included in a published review or article, no part of this book may be reproduced or transmitted in any form or by any means or media of any kind, including but not limited to photocopying, recording, or any form of information storage and retrieval, without written permission from the author.

Published and Printed in the United States of America

ISBN 0-9705832-8-1

Table of Contents

Author's Preface vii
Writing a Book and What's the Differences
Between Ultimate Diet Secrets and
Ultimate Diet Secrets Lite ix
Scientific References xiv

Chapter 1 1
How Obesity Changed a Young Boy's Life 1
Structure of This Book 7

Chapter 2 11
Ultimate Secret of Weight Control 11
Purported Success From Weight Loss
Programs is a Myth; It's Actually a Great Failure 17
The Energy Balance Equation 19
Calories Do Count 20

Chapter 3 23
Establishing the Basic Numbers 23
What's a Calorie? How Do We Measure It? 24
Determining Metabolic Rate 27
Resting Metabolic Rate 28
Calculating Your Own Resting Metabolic Rate 30
Thermic Effect of Food 33
Total Daily Energy Expenditure (TDEE) 33
Accurate Determination of Total Daily
Energy Expenditure (TDEE) 38
Calculating Calorie Needs by Eating Food 38
Two More Calculations 43
Energy-In/Energy-Out 45

Chapter 4 50
Growing Up in the Fitness Revolution 50

Chapter 5 63
Learning How to Take Control of My Body 63

Chapter 6 73
How Weight Loss (and Gain) Affect Body Composition 73
Weight Gain 79

Table of Contents

Does Becoming Overweight or Obese
Increase Calorie Needs? 81
Weight Loss 82
Lean Body Mass Changes 83
Water Losses 88
Changes in Body Composition 90
Energy Partitioning 92
How the Body's Metabolism Adapts to
Dieting and Weight Loss 95
Energy Partitioning 92
Metabolic Adaptations 94
How the Body's Metabolism Adapts
to Dieting and Weight Loss 95
What are the Effects of Overfeeding 102
Set-Point Theory of Bodyweight 104
How Do Changes in Food Intake Affect
the Two Main Parts of Calorie Burn? 106
You Must Make Adjustments When Losing Weight:
What Type of Adjustments Must You Make
in Response to Metabolic Adaptations
from Weight Loss? 113
What is the Mechanism Behind "Post-Starvation
Obesity?" 119

Chapter 7 126
The Power of Eating the Right Type of Food 126
How We Define Diet Composition 128
Unraveling the Diet Composition Mystery 130
My Conversion 130
Carbohydrate-to-Fat Conversion 133

Chapter 8 138
Why Low-Fat Diets Don't Work 138
Evidence About Low-fat Diets and Weight Loss 139
Low-fat Mania Overtakes the Country 142
"But Fat Has Twice as Many Calories
per Gram vs. Carbohydrate. Eat Fat and
You Eat Two Times More Calories,"
say the Low-fat Proponents 143

Chapter 9 145
The Complete Scoop on the Low-Carbohydrate Diet 145
History of the Low-Carbohydrate Diet 145
The Ketone Story 146
Fat is the Preferred Fuel of the Body
-- Not Carbohydrate 149
How the Body "Burns" Food 150
Body Composition Changes: Low-Carbohydrate
vs. Low-Fat 151
Why Do Low-Carbohydrate Dieters Lose More
Bodyweight than High-Carbohydrate Dieters? 154
Insulin Increases Eating and Fat Storage 158
How Low Do Carbohydrate Grams Have to Go? 160
How the Low-Carbohydrate Diet Works Metabolically ... 162

Chapter 10 165
Dietary Control of Appetite and Hunger 165
Energy-Partitioning and Food Intake 165
The Relationship Between Fat and Carbohydrate
Metabolism Determines Food Intake 168

Chapter 11 172
Crushing the Criticism Against
the Low-Carbohydrate Diet 172
Challenges to the Low-Carbohydrate Diet 172
The First Major Attacks 174
The Critics' Claims 175
Criticism: Calories Don't Count 176
Weight Loss, Appetite, and Hunger 177
The Nutrition Council's Complaints 178
Saturated Fats, Cholesterol, Triglycerides,
and Coronary Heart Disease 179
Ketosis 180
Uric Acid 181
Fatigue 182
Dizziness 183
Obesity: Diet Composition 183
Eggs 184
The Council Bangs the Gavel 185
Correcting the Errors -- On Both Sides 185
Kidney Harm 186

Table of Contents

Summary 187

Chapter 12 188
Completing My Understanding of the Energy
Balance Equation 188
The Eskimo Diet and Vilhjalmur Stefansson 190
My Own Experiments with Pemmican
and the All-Meat Diet 191
The Caltrac 192
The Final "Imprinting" of the Energy Balance Equation .. 194

Chapter 13 196
The Importance of Physical Activity
to Bodyweight Control 196
Do Physical Activity and Exercise Contribute
to Reducing Bodyweight and Body Fat? 197
The Roundtable's Conclusions and Other
Reviewers Put in Their Two Cents 198
Low Levels of Physical Activity
Contribute to Overweight 199
Settling the Confusion 201
Description of the Exercise Prescription 202
What Type of Exercise Should You Do? 204
How Exercise and Activity Affect What
You Weigh and What You Eat 205
What's the Minimum Level of Physical Activity
to Keep You Out of the Inactive Zone? 208
How Many Calories Must We Burn
to Control Bodyweight? 209
Reviewing the Modern-Day Re-Examination
of the Mayer Hypothesis 212
How Much Physical Activity Do We Need
to Lose Weight and Maintain the Loss? 214
What's the Cause of Obesity? 216

Chapter 14 218
What Changes Can You Expect
From Increased Physical Activity? 218
What Type of Exercise Should You Do? 220
Resistance Training 221
Exercise Increases Metabolic Rates:

Myth's Triumph Over Truth 225
The Differences in Metabolism Between
Fat and Muscle 228

Chapter 15 232
Putting the Program Together & Dr. Ellis's
100/100 Plan 232
Dr. Ellis's 100/100 Plan 234
Why Dr. Ellis's 100/100 Plan Works
Where Others Won't 236
Step by Step Approach to Using
Dr. Ellis's 100/100 Plan 237
Behavior Modification 243
Maintenance of Weight Loss 244

Chapter 16 250
Dr. Ellis's Version of the Low-Carbohydrate Diet 250
How Much Carbohydrate? 250
What to Do After Reaching Your Weight Loss Goal 253
"Hitting-the-Wall" or Reaching a Plateau in Weight Loss
Before Reaching Your Weight Loss Goals 253
There is a <u>Big</u> Missing Ingredient in the
Dietary Approach to Weight Loss: for both Low-Fat
<u>and</u> Low-Carbohydrate Dietary Protocols 256
Why Follow the Ellis Version of the
Low-Carbohydrate Diet? 257
How to Follow the Ellis Version of the
Low-Carbohydrate Diet 260
Carbohydrate Grams in Foods and
a Sample One Week Menu 265
Carbohydrate Content of Common Foods 268

Chapter 17 276
The Science Underlying Dr. Ellis's Weight Loss Plan 276
Predictability of Changes in Bodyweight
and Its Functions 278
Changes in Body Composition 282
Why the Focus on Diet, Alone, Doesn't Work 284
What's the First Response of the
Body to Calorie Restriction? 284
Metabolic Control of Food Intake

I heard the kitchen door close, followed a minute or two later by the door closing on our old gray Packard. I kneeled on the top of the metal radiator cover and peered out my front bedroom window, staring down onto the driveway. I watched the car back down the driveway and then slowly turn onto Glenwood Avenue.

I could almost hear the click of the automatic gearshift lever as it slipped into forward. The Packard began to move slowly up the street; it was still cool enough that the exhaust fumes turned into a billowing cloud that early morning. We'd logged a lot of miles in that car, and I felt almost as sad seeing the old car disappear up the street as I felt seeing my father disappear out of our lives.

I had no idea about what was to come. What do you know about the future at the age of 12? What would be the aftershock of his leaving? These aren't questions that I thought about at the time. It would be nice to be free of the beatings, the screaming, the tearing apart of the house. And Christmas Eve, for once, might prove to be a joyous occasion.

One year, he arrived home from work five hours late. He was drunk, usual for a Christmas Eve; I remember many. He sat my mother and me on the couch, her on one side and me on the other. Putting his arms around us, he held us captive for the next several hours, verbally torturing us. I didn't even think of fighting back for fear of something worse.

There was a time several years earlier, when he screamed at my mother. I moved between her and my father and told him to leave her alone. With that, he started screaming at me, slapping me repeatedly across the face.

I learned then to avoid his wrath.

and How Diet Composition Drives It 287
Metabolic Adaptations 290

Chapter 18 292
How I Put All the Elements Together
for the Winning Plan 292
Writing the Book 292
Those Damned Metabolic Adaptations Strike 294
I Go Off the Edge Once Again 298
How to Meet My Goals Was Becoming a Problem 302
Decreasing Calorie Needs
From Metabolic Adaptations 305
Stimulating Thermogenesis Through Everyday Drugs.... 309
All the Tools I Put Together 313
Focusing on the Major Issue Related
to Bodyweight Regulation 314
A Solution to the Problem of Under-Reporting 316
Where Do I Go From Here? 320

Index 322

Author's Preface

"Burn More Fat" exhorts the cover of the Fitness magazine stacked among the other magazines on the convenience store rack.

This is the very same message blaring out from all sorts of magazine covers and TV ads and from the lips of the "so-called experts." It seems to be the new mantra for weight loss success. Everyone has some exclusive new method to ramp-up people's metabolisms. It all sounds so easy: Just follow the procedures discussed and, voila, up goes the metabolic rate and fat just "melts" off your body.

I've got a question? Since there are so many articles and so many tips and so many books about how to ramp-up one's metabolism and since it's so easy to do, why are so many people so fat?

It's impossible for anyone to miss or to be unaware of this message; it's everywhere. Surely people are embarking upon these programs since they are, after all, **so very easy?** Anyone can do the touted program and anyone can succeed, **with no effort**, we're told.

The claim in this message must work, don't you think? Everyone, including many doctors, agrees that upping the metabolism is the way to go if we want to "melt" the fat off our bodies. The message delivery people tell us exactly what steps to take to succeed and how easy it is to succeed.

Is it?

The truth? Regrettably, no, it's not. There must be another cause, then, for the overweight epidemic because people are really being bombarded with this message.

Author's Preface

You realize, of course, that all this theorizing isn't working.

Why isn't it working? What could be the reason?

The answer is very simple, actually.

For all its seeming science, the message is a **total lie**.

It's false.

It won't work.

You're being "had" every day.

Did you ever take the time to add up how much money you've spent on products and promises, reading and believing from each the same message, over and over again, just repackaged in another "so-called expert's" words?

You'd file for bankruptcy if you could calculate how much you'd spent.

OK, why another weight loss book? It's because everything on the market doesn't work: all those "Establishment" plans concocted by the scientific and medical people, all the "radical plans," all the plans based on one idea or another, the pet theory of one author or another. They don't teach you anything. Why?

They all share a common feature: they promote misinformation, or incomplete information, or a combination of the two. **And that's true for every one of them.**

Why, I wondered, was everything out there filled with misinformation? Had no one ever taken the time to truly understand and analyze how weight loss and weight control actually work?

The answer was, no, they hadn't. But I had. I realized then that no one possessed the training or the breadth of background and experience to see their mistakes.

I knew that all of the various program designers were thought to be the "top dietary experts" in the country, and yet, even they hadn't figured out the facts.

It finally clicked and I realized that I knew more than any of the millionaire best-selling authors and other scientists about weight loss and weight control.

I realized that from all my efforts in so many diverse disciplines I'd gained a level of expertise that exceeded that of others. I understood how it all worked.

I'd spent years studying exactly how the body worked and I knew that there were unbreakable rules that dictated bodyweight control. No one else seems to have figured this out. Once you know the rules, you have absolute control. People don't know this; they think it's all just uncontrolled; a Wild West show with no rules.

Writing a Book and What's the Differences Between **Ultimate Diet Secrets** and **Ultimate Diet Secrets Lite**?

In **Ultimate Diet Secrets** (my BIG 600-page book), I described the process that I went through to produce it. I knew what I wanted to write and that was the complete 100% story about bodyweight regulation, something that no one had ever done before. I knew my book would not be "just another diet book."

I hired book shepherds after I completed the book and they all said that people would not buy a $60, 600-page, 8½ x 11 book weighing 4 pounds. I disagreed and believed that they would when they realized what I had done. I also knew that the NY publishers would slash my book down to a mass-market offering whose size and

Author's Preface

price were competitive with other books in its class, although my book was in a class by itself.

UDS, inarguably, wasn't like anything ever offered before. I knew this and my readers knew this; something I learned during the first three months after I published my book. I also learned that there was a big gap between "a reader" and a "not-yet-a-reader." I now understood that I was right and my book shepherds were wrong; I also understood that I was wrong and the shepherds were right too. It all depended upon whether or not one was a reader. If not, then standard buyer resistance intervened as the shepherds had said.

Late in November 2002, I decided to break UDS down into each individual chapter and offer the content as downloadable e-chapters that one could buy from my web site. The plan was to make entry into my content inexpensive and have someone become my reader. I knew that after one saw what I offered, something so different than all the weight loss misinformation out there, that he would then want the whole book. I knew size and price would no longer be a barrier.

People would realize that my book was unlike anything ever produced on this topic in the past. They would realize that they now possessed the encyclopedia of bodyweight regulation. How did I know this? My readers had told me so. One reader told me that "my book was insanely under-priced" and another said "I would pay 10 times the $65 for all the information."

In late November of 2002, Art Carey, a journalist with the *Philadelphia Inquirer*, wrote an article about my new book. Art writes a health and fitness column that appears regularly every Monday and my article appeared the Monday after Thanksgiving. Amazingly, just one week after the article appeared, Art called me and wanted to do a second piece about the chapter I wrote describing the myth behind the idea that increasing muscle mass through weight training increases one's calorie burn at rest.

Clearly, Art understood what I'd written. I was tearing apart a whole industry that's riddled with misinformation. And, I was smashing the myths appearing across multiple aspects of several intertwined industries, including the weight loss industry and the fitness, health, sports, and exercise/workout industries too. And, I was providing SOLUTIONS. No one had the expertise to do what I had done in my book and each and every reader knew this.

I was still wrestling with the possibility of getting a publisher and going through the process of getting my book into bookstores. I realized that any publisher would gut my book. I was, however, thinking about a preemptive strike and finding an editor who knew how to edit according to the requirements of the NY publishing houses.

On Christmas Eve 2002, I met with a company who was interested in promoting my book and using its guidelines to run a promotional weight loss class. They wanted to put the book into each of their 10 fitness store locations. We discussed the process by which the store operators would promote the book and the company owner said the only issue she thought that might be a problem was the $60 price tag.

By this time, I was pretty sick of hearing about the price of the book being too steep. I had, however, made steps to overcome this objection by offering the e-chapters. This presentation, unfortunately, would not solve the price issue at the stores, nor the issues related to price and size that the publishers would complain about. One of my readers had made a comment about "taming that monster UDS."

Author's Preface

As I left the meeting, I thought, "who better than me to do the editing process." Art Carey and I had discussed editing as he was also an experienced editor as well as a journalist. He had coined the term, "sweating-the-book-down," a term that I embraced. Upon arriving home on Christmas Eve, I began the process of "sweating-down" my big UDS. Since UDS was a book that covered all aspects of bodyweight regulation and nutrition, it had several chapters that occupied many pages that could be removed without impacting the teaching of the process of bodyweight regulation. If readers wanted these chapters later on to enhance their knowledge, then they would still be available. Nothing would be canned or deleted into oblivion. And, big UDS would continue to be a part of my offerings. Each and every word that I wrote would continue to live; I took solace in knowing this.

After knocking out a few chapters, my strategy became clear. I focused on two main actions. First, I had written 7 chapters as autobiography chapters. In these chapters, I told the story about how I learned every issue related to bodyweight regulation. People had been questioning why there was some person's autobiography in a weight control book. These chapters, however, worked; the majority of my readers told me so; only a small number didn't. But, nonetheless, out went the majority of them. Again, they would still live, but not in the pages of **Ultimate Diet Secrets Lite**. I didn't strip all of them out because I knew that some of my weight loss experiences would benefit my readers during their own process of losing weight.

Second, I had written my book as a "How To" book but I also included a detailed "Why" for every "How To." If I made a point, I wanted my readers to know exactly why I had come to that conclusion. This led to a considerable amount of scientific explanation (in terms anyone could understand -- I made sure of that -- I used MS Word which lets you check the grade level of the writing, and mine was at the 8th-10th grade level even with all the science). And my editor was a master at making my writing easy to follow.

I figured that for every page of "How To" there was one page of "Story/Autobiography" and one page of "Why." Out they went. I was ruthless in my editing work, twelve hours alone on Christmas day. My family wondered what had happened to me but I'd sort of been gone during the 3-year book-making process anyway so this was nothing out of the ordinary.

I had really fleshed UDS out and now I was paring down the flesh. UDS was, appropriately, on a post-holiday diet. My daughter suggested UDS Fat Free as a name but since I love fat and know that the whole low-fat diet scam is a mistake, I couldn't go that way.

After paring it back, I dropped the font size one notch and changed the paper size to 5½ x 8½, standard for many books today. I did a second go-round on the 26th of December, continuing my ruthless deleting. It didn't bother me too much because I knew I could still offer all of my content in a multitude of ways. My readers now had choices and I knew that I could meet the reading and buying needs of any person.

When I finished, I realized I could've never written UDS Lite first; Lite could've arisen only out of the beauty that was UDS. I like the result. All of the great content and 100% of all of the weight loss facts are still in UDS Lite. And how much did I delete? UDS Lite is now equal to about 175 letter sized pages. In other words, I cut out about 425 pages from the original 600-page UDS. Maybe 70 pages were accounted for by dropping the font size from 12 points to 11 points.

Well, that's enough. Too much rambling and I'll be back to 600-pages! If you need to know, all of the details

Author's Preface

about big UDS are on my web site and you can easily find out what topics were deleted. Within the text remaining, various paragraphs were slashed and the only way you would know which ones would be through comparing. This, I believe, would be a waste of your time. Just remember, if you need every "Why" for each "How To," and if you want the points/counterpoints to any "How To," and if you want my whole "Story," and if you want more details about nutrition, then UDS Big is for you. For example, I deleted an enormous chapter that's an expose about the major diet plans on the market, particularly a complete dismantling of the Atkins' diet. But, that chapter can be purchased by itself as an e-chapter, so it's still available, as are all the others.

In brief, thanks to Laurie, Devyn, and Chase, my family, and my dear friend, mentor, and editor, Dr. Al Thomas for his insights and fine-tuning of my work.

Scientific References

I've often been asked for a list of the references that stand behind my work. Here's my position. Those references are my proprietary work product collected through an unceasing effort stemming back almost 30 years. If someone wants to verify my writing, he must first be able to read the scientific research papers. So providing them for the average lay reader is of no value. If a reader has the training to read the research, then he also has the training to go find it. I provide enough references for names of researchers and topics for anyone trained in the art to do their own work effort and collect papers on the many topics I discuss. But, I suggest that you don't waste your time as everything in this book is true and correct. The bulk of the research content is in the big book and far less is in UDS Lite since I removed so many "Whys." Enjoy.

Gregory Ellis, PhD, CNS   January 2, 2003

Chapter 1

How Obesity Changed a Young Boy's Life

Although it was midsummer, the early morning hours were still cool. On this particular day in July, I woke early, not so much from movement in the house as from sadness that this was the day my father was going to leave -- permanently. I didn't leave my room to say goodbye because even though I didn't want him to leave, I knew he had to go.

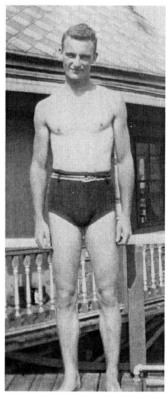

It had been a tumultuous 12 years. My mother had told me that it was painful for her and my brother even before I was born in 1947. I'd lived my childhood in a classic dysfunctional family, filled with the best of times, and the worst of times.

My father was a big man, an impressive man. He was six-foot-four, 240 pounds, and damn good-looking. He had an extraordinary personality, at least to people outside the family, one that matched his physical prowess. He'd been a star athlete in high school during the early 1930's. I still have a picture of him without a shirt; he was razor lean, with chiseled abdominal muscles.

How Obesity Changed a Young Boy's Life

His influence over me had been powerful. As a small boy, I was impressed by his athletic stories, and they seemed all the more real when I looked up at the man in all his muscle. I knew that the tales of his exploits were true. In those days, he was bigger than anyone else, bigger than life, and he had the newspaper clippings to prove it. Old varsity letters, athletic sweaters, certificates of achievement, trophies, and medals filled a half-dozen crumbling cardboard boxes.

I remember sitting on his bed on Saturday mornings, a cup of coffee on the nightstand, next to the ever-present ashtray and unfiltered Chesterfield cigarettes. Smoke rose in gentle circles from the slowly burning tobacco. As much as I detest cigarette smoke today, there are still times when I find the smell almost seductive, bathing me in warm feelings.

The big man, Ches Ellis, was a drunk, and the whole family -- my mother, my brother, and I -- was never spared from the rages burning within this troubled man. One moment our relationship with him was one of laughter and joy; the next moment, we'd find ourselves running for our lives, doing anything to avoid the beating that could happen to anyone one of us, at anytime. I was usually more successful at hiding than my brother.

My father did, however, stimulate my interest in sports and athletics. This, of course, wasn't hard to accomplish in the postwar America of the mid- to late-1950's. At that time, TV was brand-new. In fact, when my father purchased our TV set, we became the proud owners of the first one on our block. During my childhood, there were only three stations to watch, so sitting in front of a TV tube all day long was far less tempting than it is to today's kids.

● ●

How Obesity Changed a Young Boy's Life

In 1960, it was still unusual to be the child of a divorced family. My response to the breakup of my family was to eat, and that's exactly what I did. I must have eaten a lot of food because in a short time I'd gained 60 pounds. During the seventh-grade football season, I weighed slightly less than 127 pounds, the team's upper weight limit. By late the next fall, I had fattened up enormously, tipping the scales at 185 pounds. My height, however, had not increased: I remained the same 5 feet 5 inches that I had been at the end of seventh-grade. The difference was that my body had ballooned, front to back and side-to-side; I had come to occupy a lot of space. I was not a handsome sight.

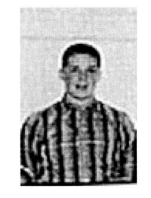

The emotional abuse meted out by my classmates was unbearable. My new nickname was "fat ass." I burrowed into a shell of fat and avoided contact with them and with life.

Up until that time, excess body fat had never been a problem for me. In fact, I was a well built young boy. At an early age, before the onset of my obesity, I'd become interested in building muscles.

Like most young boys, I'd coax an older, more muscular boy to "make a muscle," and then my friends and I would chirp with glee and grab onto that bulging arm, wrapping our hands around it. We lifted our legs off the ground to test how long this strong man could hold our weight. This was always great fun, enjoyed as much by the admired strong man as it was by my pals and me.

As my obesity increased, my health problems mounted. By the winter of 8th grade, my scalp and neck broke out in a multitude of festering, oozing, open sores. My family physician described the disease as impetigo. By the early spring, I'd broken out in another disease called pityriasis rosea. In both cases, I was given antibiotics. I also became plagued with an intractable cough, brought on by activity. It was unrelenting and choking.

Then, the pounding headaches came. With every step that I took, my head throbbed. I felt as though it would explode. Because I was in great pain, I made yet another return visit to the physician's office. He promptly diagnosed me with high blood pressure. The numbers were frightening, dangerously high, 180/110. My physician immediately placed me on blood pressure-lowering medication, at age twelve.

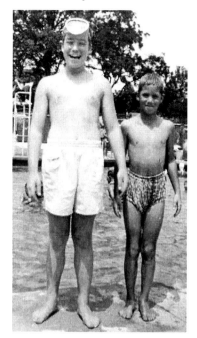

Rob, my older brother, and lean Greg before I got fat after my parent's divorce. A cute little guy who had no idea what was in store for him.

My troubles were mounting, both physically and emotionally. I was no longer participating in sports and was beset with a rash of diseases. These included obesity, skin disease, high blood pressure, and emotional/social problems.

\d become so fat and weak that I could no longer
.in even one push-up. I had also acquired a set of
"bitch-tits" (gynecomastia), most likely a side effect of my
diseased state. In addition to all of these problems, the
skin covering my shoulders and pectoral muscles began
to tear. This was the result of my rapidly increasing mass
of fat. These areas of my body became covered with
stretch marks: reddened slits where the superficial layer
of skin had split. This left many 1- to 2-inch-long scars
in the skin. Faint scars remain today, reminders of this
horrible time.

I was suffering and didn't know what to do about my
problems. No one was there to offer me any guidance.

The physician just drugged me. I was a social outcast
as a child from a parentally divorced family. I was both
obese and diseased. My mother had nothing to offer
because she was suffering, herself, while trying to raise
two teenage boys as a single parent with little money.
The doctor offered no advice because he knew nothing
about weight control. He surely didn't associate my
obesity with my emotional troubles and my diseases.
Even today, most physicians don't discuss weight control
with their patients. This was, and is, especially true
when the patient is a young boy.

●●●●●●●●●●●●●●●●●●●●●●●●●●

I plotted my course and knew that I had my work cut
out for me: I was fat, very fat. At the time, all I knew was
that I was fat, but not merely in the medical or scientific
sense. I was a fat person who'd become a social outcast.

Looking back, armed with modern measuring tools, I
can calculate exactly how fat I was in comparison with
standard measures of body fatness. Using the only two
measurements that I have in my personal file, my height
and weight, I've calculated my Body Mass Index during

those years. In simple terms, this is a measure of how much weight one's body carries per unit of height. This is similar to the Metropolitan Weight Scale that has been used for many years, but more efficient than that now-outdated scale.

My Body Mass Index at 5 feet, 5 inches and a weight of 185 pounds was 30.8. For a 12-year-old boy, the healthy range is between 18-21. An Index of 26 (not 30 plus) places a boy in the very fat range: at the 97th percentile for overweight. Because of the health risks associated with obesity, it's no surprise that I was suffering from diseases. Using the same method to calculate my Index during the previous year, at 5 feet, 5 inches and 127 pounds, my value was 21.2, perfectly in the normal range.

Structure of This Book

In my quest to solve my own obesity problem, I've tried, during the last four decades, every available weight loss method. The process that I went through is similar to the one that anyone interested in losing weight pursues.

I ventured down many dead-end streets. There are so many competing theories, and because of our inability to decipher whether any of these theories is effective, we endlessly try out a multitude of advertised and marketed weight loss and weight control programs. Far more often than not, the method we choose fails, and then we're off, yet again, on a never-ending search for the golden fleece of weight control.

Currently, more than 60% of our population suffers from an overweight condition. I believe, in reality, this is an underestimate.

How Obesity Changed a Young Boy's Life

It's imperative for all of us to realize that the weight control problem can be solved. Through my long study and experimentation, I've resolved the questions related to weight control. There are scientifically sound answers and methods that help people attain their goals. Unfortunately, as stated, it's difficult for any one person, unaided, to unearth these solutions. It's my goal, then, to hook you up with a set of blinders, permitting you to reach your goal, weight control, without all the marketplace's distractions.

Unfortunately, I approached weight control in the same way that it was presented to me, in pieces. That's undoubtedly how it has been presented to you: with each piece being magnified so as to represent the whole, complex solution to your overweight, obesity, and "I'm-too-fat condition": the one technique or strategy that will solve your problem.

It's easy to sell you weight loss in a bottle, but it's harder to sell an integrated program made up of many different parts, a program whose every part is absolutely required to help you achieve your goals.

Weight control in animals is a highly regulated biological function. As such, biological Laws control our weight and its composition. These Laws are inviolate: they operate in each and every one of us. We are all subject to the same Laws. Once understood, you finally become the master of your weight (and body).

Ultimate Diet Secrets are methods of weight control providing a unique opportunity for you to, at last, gain the upper hand at weight control. Using my methods helps us understand and control every aspect of the weight loss and weight control equation. This program emphasizes a complete understanding of the complex nature of weight control, and it provides each individual the means of control required to achieve success. Many popular weight control programs de-emphasize the importance of calculating various parts of the weight loss and weight control equation. Whole schools, within the market-driven sector and the scientific community, have devised soft-peddled approaches that relieve fat-laden persons of any personal responsibility for their overweight condition.

We now know that bodyweight is precisely controlled by in-born regulatory mechanisms. The efforts of a legion of scientific researchers during the last 150 years have uncovered the guiding principles of weight control. These principles give us meticulous control over bodyweight regulation. When applied, they effect specific responses that solve the weight problem.

I'm going to lead you, here, step-by-step, through the process of gaining complete and absolute control over your weight and body composition. The specific concepts that I'll cover have been hard-won for me personally. They will, however, improve your chances of success while minimizing your failures.

My program is a comprehensive one. It identifies all aspects of the weight loss and weight control equation. It derails many current ideas and programs as myths and falsehoods. My program is not shortsighted, nor is it limited to only a few pieces of the puzzle. When you finish this book, you'll understand every aspect of how to lose and control your weight. It took me close to 45 years to understand fully the essentials of weight loss and weight control. I wish that it hadn't proved to be such a formidable task; it won't be for you.

Until now, it's been difficult to acquire and master the fundamental concepts of weight control. The blame for this confusion falls upon the purveyors of products and services for-profit. The blame also falls upon our medical and scientific community which often appear just as confused as the public and the marketers. These so-called scientists have been hamstrung by their own biases and by their personal inexperience.

Many of the existing approaches are far too limited. My program is the product of my exhaustive research and personal experience. Through painful experience, I learned the techniques required to solve the overweight condition and to optimize body shape and body composition to any desired degree.

First, I'm going to teach you what I actually learned last, many years after trying all the different "plans" out there, suffering through the endless ideas promoted by thousands of authors and pundits who, unwittingly, confuse us with so many false ideas. For example, I just read a review of a new book by a self-proclaimed fitness guru who argues that we should throw away our cardiovascular equipment because, like hormone therapy, it's not getting the job done. He argues for building muscle through strength training as the only way to go because "lean muscle tissue burns more calories than fat." That's true but it's misleading and irrelevant. He says that many problems are thwarting Americans who want to drop pounds because chaotic theories muddle the field. He's right. And, his theories are at the top of the list of theories that muddle. I will dig you out of all the **CONFUSION**.

I will tell some of this story, as I've already done in this chapter, by describing my own life's highway. You'll see how I suffered just as you have. In my 600-page book, my autobiography represents a significant proportion of those pages. It tells a story and it teaches. Here, in UDS Lite, I've removed much of that story, keeping that which I believe will add to your learning experience. I don't think it'll bore you and I think you'll say, "That happened to me too and now I know exactly where I went wrong."

Chapter 2

Ultimate Secret of Weight Control

Physicists today are attempting to construct a theory capable of explaining everything. Albert Einstein's physics was quite different from the laws of physics established by Newton in the late 1600's. Newtonian physics was applicable to the large-scale world, but the physics of Einstein concerned the sub-atomic realm.

Bodyweight control follows Newtonian Laws which were formulated several hundred years before Albert Einstein was born. Einstein's physics isn't a solution to our overweight condition. We won't find the answers to weight control by using principles that explain Einstein's sub-atomic world.

All living cells and organisms must perform work to stay alive, to grow, and to reproduce. A fundamental function of each cell is the ability to extract energy from different chemical sources. The cell, then, uses this energy to perform biological work.

Our bodies have a very sophisticated system for converting one form of energy to another and Nature provides energy for human beings in various forms. Chemical energy stored in food provides the energy from which our body makes its complex molecules, the stuff of our flesh. Complex molecules have a highly ordered structure and the body manufactures these molecules from simple compounds. It converts the chemical energy contained in nature's fuels into electrical activity, motion, and heat.

We've known for centuries that chemicals provide the material for energy production and a large volume of scientific research uncovered the process by which cells extract and use this energy.

Antoine Lavoisier (1743-1794) understood that animals converted chemical fuels into work and heat. Lavoisier stated, "This fire stolen from heaven, this torch of Prometheus, does not only represent an ingenious and poetic idea, it is a faithful picture of the operations of nature, at least for animals that breathe; one may therefore say, with the ancients, that the torch of life lights itself at the moment the infant breathes for the first time, and it does not extinguish itself except at death."

Scientists have uncovered the processes by which the body converts chemical fuels into work, heat, and life. Their studies have demonstrated the fascinating mechanisms by which organisms convert food to fuel. This is understood down to the smallest unit of the body, the gene. The key fact from these studies is that energy conversions obey **absolutely** the same physical Laws governing all natural processes.

Therefore, it's essential that any individual interested in controlling his bodyweight understand these Laws of Nature. He must understand these Laws of the flow of energy in and out of our bodies.

Newton's Laws of Thermodynamics, therefore, govern biological energy conversions. These Laws, first codified in the 19th century, include both the First and the Second Law of Thermodynamics. The First Law is the principle of the Conservation of Energy. It states that, in any physical or chemical change, the total amount of energy in the universe remains constant, although the form of the energy may change. The Second Law states that the universe always tends toward more and more disorder. This is called entropy, and as a function of all natural processes, this Law implies that the disorder of the universe increases.

Our bodies are a collection of complex molecules which are much more organized than the materials from which they have sprung. The body attempts to maintain itself by producing order, fighting entropy or the tendency of the body to become disordered. To do so, however, requires putting energy into the system. At the same time, however, the system releases disorder into the environment. These two actions are consistent with the Second Law of Thermodynamics.

Every part of the body -- including such highly developed systems as the muscular system, the nervous system, and the circulatory system -- operates under the Laws. These Laws also operate within the individual cell: within the mitochondrion, the gene, and DNA.

We can conclude from the above explanation that we are **absolutely obligated** to live under the well-defined Laws of Thermodynamics.

No one can escape; no one is above the Laws.

In simple words, then, the calories one consumes must equal the calories one burns for bodyweight to remain constant. If one consumes more than he burns, he gains weight. If one consumes less than he burns, he loses weight. The best way to state this is, **Calories Do Count!**

This, then, is the first principle. Its absolute understanding is essential to bodyweight maintenance and regulation.

Failure to understand the operation of the Laws causes the extreme frustration suffered by millions of people plagued by overweight and obesity and of those already fit and in shape who want to look even better.

Without an understanding of these guiding principles, we are prey to the hucksters with all their pills and potions and quick-weight loss schemes.

Instead, armed with these guiding principles, we can ward off the huckster's attack.

This failure to understand the Laws, however, is as much a problem with the scientific community as it is with the public. Publications appearing in scientific journals as recently as the late 1990's continue to say that obese persons are beyond the control and power of the Laws. So does Dr. Robert Atkins, mistakenly.

These unscientific conclusions were reached by these scientists and pseudo-scientists because of the difficulty of making accurate measurements and interpretations. Changes in bodyweight, precipitated by some intervention, reflect changes in various body compartments: the body's fat content, its muscle and organ content, and its water weight.

Another cause of science's continued misinterpretation is its failure to thoroughly investigate the historical research record which has consistently demonstrated the **ironclad** action of the Laws. Early research, occurring in 1866, demonstrated that there was an exact balance between the amount of oxygen consumed by a starving man and the amount of fat and protein burned by his body: the calories consumed matched those that burned.

The validity of the Laws of Thermodynamics for animal metabolism is universally accepted among scientists. But, amazingly, however, even today, there are multitudes of purveyors of weight loss pills and regimens who argue against the existence of these guiding principles.

That obesity is so prevalent can be directly attributed to the many "scientists" and dietary frauds who have failed to help people understand these guiding principles. They have, instead, attempted to profit through the sales of their miraculous, no-effort, free-lunch weight loss plans.

It follows, then, that bodyweight maintenance is dictated by the Laws: the calorie value of the food **consumed** and **used** by the body must, therefore, be **equal** to the body's **energy expenditure** for bodyweight to remain constant. Therefore, the calorie value of food must be equal to the calories the body uses to perform work and to create heat that's lost to the environment for bodyweight to remain constant.

For an individual undergoing a weight loss regimen, the lost weight contains a specific calorie value. We can calculate it. We must be careful, though, because several variables **affect** this calculation. I will cover these later. The **failure** to lose weight is a common characteristic shared by many millions of people **attempting** to lose weight. The other major problem is that people often lose less weight than predicted.

Often the measured weight loss and its calculated calorie value disagree with an estimate of the calorie burn of the individual. There are two possibilities, 1) we must suspect an error in the calculation of the amount of calories consumed and 2) Metabolic Adaptations occur in response to weight loss. There are no other possibilities according to the Laws. Later, I will detail the affects of Metabolic Adaptations and how they create confusion and frustration in weight loss efforts.

Unfortunately, blame for these discrepancies falls upon some factor other than careless and dishonest calorie counting. This opens the door to the multitude of false ideas about how to control weight, leading ultimately to mass confusion. Failure and frustration follow. Even those making the sincerest attempts to control weight are confronted with failures and frustrations.

There is probably no part of human nutrition surrounded by more myths than the calorie. These myths pervade all parts of our society. And, surprisingly, they pervade our society's research community as well.

As I've described above, the techniques of measuring human energy **burning** have been available for close to 150 years. The task of precisely measuring energy **intake**, however, was, and is, extraordinarily difficult.

New measurement techniques, developed less than 20 years ago, now allow researchers to accurately determine energy use. The technique known as doubly-labeled water is extraordinarily accurate. It provides the researcher with unquestionably sound information about how many calories an individual burns. As a result of knowing how many calories a person burns, we have an objective measure, also, of the number of calories he has consumed.

This is because the First Law of Thermodynamics states that energy intake equals energy losses, plus or minus any energy stored or removed from the body. The energy stores of the body are, in fact, it's bodyweight.

When bodyweight remains constant, energy intake must **exactly** balance energy output. The ideal level of energy intake is that amount of food needed to maintain cell mass and function. At the same time, this intake should promote optimum health and longevity.

Evaluating the optimal calorie intake of an individual isn't easy. The difficulty of estimating calorie needs has led to many myths about the number of calories an individual consumes.

The results of all this misinformation and myth are America's burgeoning waistlines and behinds. The success rates for weight loss and weight maintenance are abysmal.

Purported Success From Weight Loss Programs is a Myth; It's Actually a Great Failure

For decades, people have dieted without success. Dieters have tried many weight loss options because there's no limit to the number of weight loss options available.

However, the result is always the same. During the first week or two, people lose 5-10 pounds. Unfortunately, this is mostly water, yet most people, astonishingly, believe that it's 100% fat. After this initial rapid weight loss, bodyweight loss slows or stops completely. Their normal-weight friends, they complain, eat all the food they want (it seems). Yet, they never gain an inch or a pound (it seems).

What is the perceived reason for the failure to lose bodyweight: a low metabolism? Or do their normal weight friends just burn calories faster?

I'm sorry to have to disabuse you as to the notion that some people can eat without consequence. They can't. Nobody can.

The truth is that you don't get enough physical activity or exercise and you eat a lot more food than you admit. Ah! So that's it; that's the answer.

Yes, it is the answer.

Finally, you have the answer.

How do I know this? Because I know the Laws. If you fail to lose weight, applying the Laws will uncover the reason for failing. This is the conclusion of many recent studies using the doubly-labeled water technique and a calorimeter.

Doubly-labeled water is a heavy isotope of water that subjects drink, and several weeks later measurements of the amount of isotope remaining in the body provide an extremely accurate measure of the body's calorie burn over the previous weeks. The calorimeter is a large, completely sealed, live-in laboratory designed to facilitate the precise measurement of food intake and calorie burn. These two methods have turned weight control research that occurred previous to the development of these techniques into chaos.

The conclusions from the studies using these measuring techniques are clearly no surprise, based on more than 100 years of research. What's surprising is that people are still trying to figure it out, as if we don't already know the answer.

The notion that there are large differences in metabolic rates just isn't true. People can no longer use this as an excuse for their weight problems; doubly-labeled water and the calorimeter don't lie.

Do we now know the secret to weight control? We sure do.

We have all been subjected to a plethora of misinformation regarding the best methods of weight control. Yet, science knows that bodyweight maintenance is contingent upon the mechanisms we've discussed in the preceding paragraphs. We must match the amount of food we consume with the amount of food we burn each day.

Nobody, anywhere, is spared from this dietary "cliché." I often sit with people to discuss a weight control program and ask them whether they know the answer to controlling their weight. Invariably, they look at me with a befuddled expression on their faces.

They are so overwhelmed with the competing weight loss choices in the marketplace that they **have absolutely no idea that bodyweight is a very precisely controlled function and acts by One Law that's operative in Every Person**.

They have no idea that they have absolute power and complete control over their bodyweight.

Their are many challenges to controlling bodyweight. The body's processing of calories modifies and affects the Laws. This increases the complexity of predicting the effects of consuming a specific **number** and **type** of calories. But, we're not yet ready for a detailed discussion about how **eating** a calorie is different from the laboratory measurement of determining the calorie value of foods. We'll get into that later on.

The Energy Balance Equation

Balancing Energy-Input (*how much you eat*) with Energy-Output (*how much you burn*)

I want, now, to finalize your understanding of the most important feature of weight control. Everything else that we do in any weight loss and weight control program is, ultimately, controlled by the Energy Balance Equation which, itself, obeys the Laws of Thermodynamics.

Finally, we get to the ***Ultimate Secret of Weight Control***. People and weight loss hucksters say that by eating a special food or taking some pill, elixir, or herbal concoction, we can melt fat from our bodies.

Forget it! It doesn't work. No one can disobey the Laws of Nature. Weight control is the **Energy Balance Equation**. Fat will not melt from the body like butter melting in a hot pan.

There are two parts to the Energy Balance Equation: what you eat and what you burn. Almost all marketed weight loss and weight control programs have one common goal: to get you to eat less than you burn.

Unfortunately, these diet programs just keep cutting what you eat and rarely worry about what you burn. They focus solely on one part of the Energy Balance Equation. In addition, if they do talk about the other part -- the number of calories that you burn -- they say "get some exercise." Exercise and increasing activity are rarely the focal points of the program -- any program.

With my program, activity and exercise comprise the focal point. Cutting calories is of secondary importance.

There are all kinds of problems with cutting calories. Moreover, the reason that weight loss and weight control programs fail to keep weight off is that they focus solely on calorie reduction, and this focus always fails. Such a plan, focused upon dieting, pays attention to only one-half of the Energy Balance Equation -- the half concerned with how much you eat.

I believe this is the wrong part to focus on.

Here is the rule of weight control: Bodyweight will not change if the calories you eat match the calories you burn. Period.

Calories Do Count

Even today, some of the leading weight loss

marketers continue to argue that calories don't count. The failure to understand that calorie balance is the **primary** consideration in regulating bodyweight is the leading reason for our burgeoning weight control problem.

Moreover, the only solution to the weight control problem is to consume fewer calories and to burn more calories. And the emphasis must be on burning more calories.

Eat more than you burn and you gain weight; eat less and you lose weight. Whatever calories you eat in excess of what you need -- whether fat, carbohydrate, or protein -- are stored as fat. It takes about 3,500 extra calories to make a pound of fat, although this varies with body fat percent, as we'll learn. Your body has a very delicate balance system to control this, and even 10 extra calories daily are stored as fat, leading to a fat increase of 1 pound each year. If this continues for 20 years, you can expect to become very fat. (This calculation is a bit simplistic and not wholly accurate. I'll explain the details to you in later, but let's get the fundamental concepts down first before delving into all of the factors that munch them up.)

This is the average increase in weight that people experience from age 25 to age 55. 100 extra calories daily is 10 pounds per year. Or, during the holiday season (Thanksgiving to New Year's Day), 500 extra calories daily give you 5 extra pounds of unwanted fat (Eat drink and be merry).

There's no way to get around the fact that taking-in 3,500 extra calories, all at once or over time, makes you gain weight. Nothing and no one can stop this from happening -- no matter what you've heard. This is a fact. And it's time for you to face it.

Conversely, when the body receives fewer calories than it burns, it takes fat from the fat stores and it burns that fat to provide the extra energy needed by the body.

There are three ways to unbalance the Energy Balance Equation and lose weight:

1) eat less than you normally burn;
2) eat what you normally eat and increase the amount you burn; and
3) do a little of both 1 and 2 by increasing what you burn and decreasing the amount you eat.

There you have it. The Ultimate Secret of Weight Control. The Secret to Losing Weight and Keeping It Off *is* the Energy Balance Equation. **And the least effective way to try to unbalance the equation is to cut calories**.

You now understand the most important fact required to lose and control weight: the Laws underlying the Energy Balance Equation.

The Laws are inviolate; everyone is subject to their power.

In a following chapter, I'll explain the calculations -- the numbers and information -- needed for you to take complete control of your weight. This is the fundamental first step. Armed with this information, you'll have a roadmap to guide your journey.

Chapter 3

Establishing the Basic Numbers

I've established that the Energy Balance Equation is the most important factor in bodyweight loss and control. Now, it's time to begin to look at the common denominator of the Energy Balance Equation -- the calorie.

Don't panic or start screaming, "Oh my God, not the calorie."

There are too many people and programs doing all they can to avoid the calorie. All types of elaborate systems exist for avoiding a confrontation with the calorie. These include color-coded cards, cutouts of different foods, point systems, and pre-packaged foods.

I've never understood this aversion to the calorie since it's the primary unit that determines our bodyweight. There are many opponents to putting the calorie at the top of the priority list. They argue that their methods of controlling food intake are less demanding than counting calories. They argue that their methods are more effective than counting calories.

I believe that downplaying the calorie's importance makes it **impossible** to effectively lose and control bodyweight. We must stand and squarely face the calorie, and until we do, we limit our chances of success in weight control. As I've stated, the main reason people downplay the importance of the calorie is because of confusion. This is true in both the public mind and in the scientific mind. This has led to a diminishment of the **primary** importance of the calorie.

Establishing the Basic Numbers

There have been many discrepancies occurring among individuals undergoing weight loss. Therefore, many people, including scientists, have claimed that the Laws of Nature don't apply to bodyweight regulation.

I've thoroughly quashed this idea. The explanation to the discrepancies is rooted in our inability to accurately measure changes resulting from weight loss. It has been difficult, until recently, to accurately determine changes in the different parts of the body from weight loss. The main body tissues undergoing change include the lean tissue (organs and muscle), fat tissue, and water.

More important, though, has been the impossibility of knowing how many calories people actually eat. Methods for accurately knowing people's food intake were only developed in 1982.

So, it's precisely for these reasons, above, that we're perplexed. It's precisely for these reasons that the Energy Balance Equation **seems** not to "work."

There are two sides to the Energy Balance Equation, Energy-In and Energy-Out. We measure them by the calculation of calories in and calories out. Therefore, the **calorie must be** the **fundamental** factor in evaluating the responses of our body to attempts to control weight.

So, instead of avoiding the calorie, we must embrace it. We must suffuse ourselves with its Power. We must enlist it as an ally instead of an enemy. Much like the aikido master, we'll use our opponent's force against him.

What's a Calorie? How Do We Measure It?

What's a calorie? It's the amount of heat required to raise the temperature of one gram of water one degree centigrade.

How do we measure it? We place a food, such as an apple, or a piece of beef, inside a small desktop-sized oven. We call this oven a bomb calorimeter. This oven operates at a very high temperature. A water jacket with a known volume surrounds the oven and a temperature gauge is in contact with the water. This allows us to accurately measure any change in the water's temperature. Now, we turn the oven on. Then we burn the food to ashes. The rise occurring in the water's temperature is a measure of the calorie content of the food. This is how we accurately measure the calories in food.

By the late 1800's through the early 1900's, many scientists contributed to figuring out the calories in most foods. This work contributed to the on-going efforts to evaluate the relationship between a human being's calorie burn and food intake.

Wilbur Atwater was one of the key players in determining the calories in foods. He also attempted to find out the calorie amount of work a man could perform in a day. He tried to relate that to the amount of food the man needed to eat. Atwater's dietary recommendations were based upon the weight of a food one should eat: the grams of protein, fat, and carbohydrate; and the ounces of liquid involved. He avoided using the calorie directly.

The physiologist, Russell Chittenden, was one of the first scientists who matched food intake to its calorie content. He used the calorie as his unit of measure. He recognized that metabolism was an issue of calorie balance. We credit Chittenden with the idea of eating based upon calories. Therefore, the idea of eating for calories isn't an old concept.

With the calorie data in hand, it should have been an easy task to solve the old problem of excess flesh, once and for all. But this balancing act didn't work out.

Establishing the Basic Numbers

Here was the problem. **Different-sized** individuals seemed to respond in a multitude of ways to eating **similar** amounts of calories.

People observed that a fat person ate like a bird. Or, so it seemed. Yet, he would gain pound after pound. The interpretation, then, was that fat people were fat because they burned their food more slowly. Or more thoroughly.

They were deemed to possess a "metabolic efficiency." They could eat small meals and become heavier. Their thin counterparts, though, it seemed, could eat endless amounts of food. And, their bodyweight never changed.

This was, and **still** is, believed to be the problem.

It was believed that thin people simply burned-off the large amounts of the food they ate. It seemed that they had a sort of "metabolic inefficiency." It was as if they were "wasting" energy.

This belief about differences in metabolic rates is, as I've stated, still prevalent today, existing at all levels of the culture.

It is, indeed, only recently that we have developed technology to solve this 100-year old riddle. We know that the measurement of food intake is very imprecise. This fact renders **useless** most of the studies, except those during the last twenty years, that evaluated this variable of weight control.

The Laws of Thermodynamics are 100% in operation. What we've discovered is that overweight people mis-report the amount of food they eat! And the fatter one becomes, the more he mis-reports.

During the last decade, we've come to understand the characteristics of under-reporters of food intake. Under-reporting increases throughout childhood and adolescence. It's more common in women than men. Smokers are more likely to under-report what they eat. Persons low in literacy and income under-report. Obese subjects and post-obese subjects (those who were obese and lost weight) under-report. Persons who carefully watch what they eat in order to avoid gaining weight under-report.

We've only learned the extent of under-reporting during the last 10-15 years.

Awareness of under-reporting has led to the development of methods to measure calorie intake. However, this is still a very complex problem. It's still easy to draw incorrect conclusions about the cause of obesity by relying on reports about the amount of food people eat, or the amounts that others "think" they ate. This is particularly true in overweight. As weight increases, so does under-reporting. Under-reporting has been the most significant limitation to understanding factors involved in the causes of obesity.

Determining Metabolic Rate

Since calories do count, we must know how to count them. Here's the first step, then, in becoming the master of your bodyweight. You must know how many calories you burn. To do this, you must understand the Energy-In and Energy-Out sides of the Energy Balance Equation. I'll now focus on the Energy-Out part of the equation. This will provide you with a complete understanding of how to calculate your calorie burn. Let's start with the calories you burn each day.

The Total Daily Energy Expenditure (TDEE) of an individual comprises three parts:
1) Resting Metabolic Rate (RMR)
2) Thermic Effect of Food (TEF)

3) Voluntary Physical Activity (PAL)

Resting Metabolic Rate

The Resting Metabolic Rate (RMR) is the obligated part of the Total Daily Energy Expenditure (TDEE). It's defined as the number of calories burned while lying still, but awake, following a 12-hour fast. The calorie burning of RMR fluctuates within a range of about 5%. RMR represents the calories burned to maintain life including nerve conduction, breathing, heart activity, muscle tone, and body temperature. In short, RMR is the calories burned to stay alive.

Again, this is the obligated part of your daily calorie burn. For most modern-day populations, RMR represents approximately 75% of the TDEE (Total Daily Energy Expenditure).

During the last 100 years there's been a remarkable amount of scientific investigation of the factors involved in RMR. There's a very strong relationship between RMR and bodyweight. This is true among human beings and other mammals with widely ranging body sizes. Of the four major parts of bodyweight -- lean tissue (organs and muscle, also known as the Lean Body Mass), fat, bone, and water -- the Lean Body Mass (LBM) is the best single predictor of RMR. It beats bodyweight, but not by a lot.

It's also well understood that RMR (Resting Metabolic Rate) is dependent upon, primarily, the size and activity of the organs. These include the brain, lungs, liver, and kidneys. They're all part of LBM, and are 60-80% of the RMR.

Muscle, although it represents 30-50% of bodyweight, is **not** a major contributor to RMR, about 20-25%. It's a minor calorie consumer when contrasted with the contribution of the organs because resting muscle burns few calories for its maintenance.

This strong relationship between RMR and LBM led to the development of mathematical formulas to predict RMR. The original formulations were published in 1919. Research during the next 40 years consistently confirmed the accuracy of the equations within +/- 5%.

Obviously, then, scientists can accurately measure RMR in a laboratory. However, the laboratory measurement of RMR is inconvenient, costly, and impractical. In lieu of making a direct measurement of RMR, we use easily obtained information about an individual to **estimate** RMR. We plug this information into a mathematical formula, crunch the numbers, and come up with a predicted RMR. This may not get us into the stadium seat as a direct measurement would, but it gets us into the ballpark.

Recent changes relative to body size and body composition, levels of physical activity, and diet led modern researchers to question the 1919 formulations. Advances in technology for measuring RMR have led to an increased number of publications reviewing the calculations of RMR. One of the outcomes of this volume of research was a verification of the relationship between RMR (Resting Metabolic Rate) and LBM (Lean Body Mass).

This strong relationship, first established in 1919, between an individual's LBM and RMR comes as a surprise to many people. In my clinical nutrition work, I've never encountered a client who believed that I could calculate his metabolism by using height, weight, sex, and age. People believe that metabolic rates vary widely among individuals of the same size. This isn't true and RMR (metabolism) varies depending on the factors I've just listed.

This belief, that people have different and widely varying metabolic rates, serves, of course, as the basis for the endless array of weight control products and programs. And because people believe calorie needs vary widely, people often don't believe that I'm telling the truth about the predictability of RMR.

Calculating Your Own Resting Metabolic Rate

Knowing that we can accurately predict RMR provides you with a golden opportunity. Calculating your own RMR is the first step in gaining absolute control over your bodyweight.

One important point: These numbers are predictions, not direct measurements. As such, they are close but not exact. They are good enough, however, to provide a baseline, a starting point. As I said, they get you into the ballpark, but don't get you into your seat.

Let's now make this first calculation. Let's build the foundation for your weight loss and weight control program. (All of the formulas that follow are available on my web site, http://www.ultimatedietsecrets.com/ by clicking a Nav tab that says **Chapter 4 Calculations**. Log on to the site, click on the page for the formulas, enter the information requested, and the program will calculate your values). If you like to do math, however, here's the formulas to make the RMR prediction:

| M | RMR= | (9.99 x weight (kg)) + (6.25 x height (cm)) − (4.92 x age) + 5 |
| F | RMR= | (9.99 x weight (kg)) + (6.25 x height (cm)) − (4.92 X age) − 161 |

You'll need to make an accurate measure of your weight and height. I'll assume that figuring out your sex and age is easy. Once you have these four pieces of information, figure out your RMR.

Convert your weight in pounds to kilograms (kg) by dividing your weight in pounds by 2.2. Convert your height in inches to centimeters (cm) by multiplying your height in inches by 2.54. Pick the appropriate formula for your sex (M = males, F = female). First do the multiplications. Follow the multiplication steps by the additions and subtractions. Once completed, you'll have an estimate of your RMR in calories a day.

These formulas are very accurate. For most people, they predict RMR within 5% of that measured in a laboratory. Some individual RMRs, however, will be miscalculated by a larger amount. In very rare instances, the miscalculation may lead to a discrepancy of 200-300 calories a day.

Most large universities have the technology to make these measurements. If you're following the program, but failing to achieve your goals, a measurement of your RMR would be the next step.

RMR can change. Two primary things change it:

1) the number of calories consumed each day (consuming either more or fewer calories)
2) changes in bodyweight leading to changes in Lean Body Mass and body fat, a topic I discuss thoroughly in the chapter on body composition and in the two chapters about Metabolic Adaptations.

Therefore, the decision to reduce calorie intake to lose weight leads to an automatic reduction in RMR. Reductions (or increases) in RMR arise from self-regulatory control mechanisms within the body.

The composition of weight loss (or gain) for any individual is approximately 75% fat and 25% LBM (Lean Body Mass). These percentages vary depending on the severity of the caloric restriction. They also depend on initial fat percent. Following a plan of severe calorie restriction (eating from 0 to 600-800 calories a day) causes losses of LBM as much as 50% of the weight loss.

I definitely don't recommend a calorie restriction of this magnitude. Big drops in RMR begin to occur when decreasing calorie intake below 1,200 a day.

For individuals who are significantly overweight, fat losses compose more of the weight loss in the initial stages than LBM (Lean Body Mass). As weight loss continues, one loses more and more LBM as a percentage of the loss.

Later on, I'll detail the specific changes in response to dieting. I'll elaborate upon weight loss caused solely by the reduction in calories consumed vs. weight loss caused solely by an increase in physical activity.

It's important to understand that it's impossible to alter RMR in any way other than described above (although some herbs can have a slight effect).

The current opinion that the acquisition of muscle tissue will significantly alter RMR is false. I'll devote a chapter to a detailed discussion of this misinformation that has strong roots in the popular culture.

● ●

In the previous section I've described the most critical part of your metabolism. This, of course, is RMR. It's that part of your calorie burn that's obligated to maintain life. We can predict RMR. And, I've shown you how we accurately predict your own RMR. This is the first step in gaining control over your bodyweight.

● ●

Thermic Effect of Food

It has been well known for a long time that the digestion of food consumes calories. In earlier times, the calories burned in the process of food digestion was called Specific Dynamic Action. The modern terminology is the Thermic Effect of Food (TEF). This part of metabolism has been explored in great detail but much confusion still remains with many unanswered questions. It's well understood that TEF accounts for about 6-10% of the Total Daily Energy Expenditure (TDEE), a small percentage of TDEE. TEF is a relatively constant figure that's not easily changed. Thus, there's no need to spend our time exploring TEF as a factor in weight control.

● ●

Total Daily Energy Expenditure (TDEE)

TDEE is the sum of the Resting Metabolic Rate (RMR), Thermic Effect of Food (TEF), and the amount of the daily physical activity level (PAL). RMR, as I've described, is the amount of calories that you burn each day to maintain life. Your body is obligated to burn this number of calories each day.

Of the three parts making up TDEE (Total Daily Energy Expenditure), PAL (Physical Activity Level) is the most variable. And it's under your control, unlike RMR. You can choose to move or not to move. To maintain a steady bodyweight requires that you eat the number of calories that's equal to your total calorie burn each day (TDEE).

For decades, scientists have tried to develop accurate methods to measure the calorie burn of human beings. Sophisticated measurements are now available and can accurately determine TDEE within about 3-4%.

Establishing the Basic Numbers

Unfortunately, this technology is too expensive to use in measuring the calorie burn for individuals. Not only is this technique expensive, the materials to run the test are hard to come by. I recently tried to have this test run on myself, unfortunately five different laboratories turned me down.

There's a worldwide effort to develop simple, inexpensive, and accurate methods for predicting TDEE. In the last decade, an enormous amount of research established the baseline values for the calorie burn of individuals. The purpose of this on-going international research project is to acquire a complete understanding of human calorie requirements.

This is important because of the worldwide increase in obesity. Because of the enormous health risks and costs involved in obesity, it's imperative that we arrive at solutions.

In 1985, the World Health Organization (WHO) expert committee on energy requirements expressed the calorie needs of adults as multiples of RMR (Resting Metabolic Rate). The index TDEE/RMR (Total Daily Energy Expenditure/Resting Metabolic Rate) serves as a method of determining physical activity level (PAL), the part of calorie burn that you control. By subtracting RMR from TDEE, we get at a number that is the calories used in physical activity (PAL).

The ratio provides a convenient way of controlling for age, sex, weight, and body composition. It also expresses the calorie needs of a wide range of people in shorthand form. The WHO set the standards for average daily calorie requirements for men. These figures are 1.55, 1.78, and 2.10 times RMR for light, moderate, or heavy occupational work, respectively. The figures established for women were 1.56, 1.64, and 1.82 times RMR.

As an example, say one's RMR (Resting Metabolic Rate) is 1,500 calories a day. For a male having a moderate level of physical activity (PAL), we multiply 1,500 times 1.78. This number is the predicted TDEE (Total Daily Energy Expenditure), 2,670 calories a day. To arrive at PAL, we subtract RMR from TDEE. This is 1,170 calories.

These ratios serve as guidelines for recommendations about an individual's calorie intake based on his calorie burn. We use these calculations to evaluate calorie intakes and calorie needs in a variety of situations.

I have, in this section, provided you with an accurate way of approximating the calories you need to eat to meet your calorie requirements. This is the value of my **Ultimate Diet Secrets** program.

Guided by the Laws, I've individualized for you an approximation of your calorie requirements. Armed with this information, you now possess your base information. Now, you can take control of your bodyweight. You are your own master.

All marketed weight loss methods **must** affect one side, or both sides, of the Energy Balance Equation to succeed. The marketers may not know this, or they may not tell you this.

The key point, though, is that **any** weight loss program **must** affect one side, or both sides, of the Energy Balance Equation if it is to succeed.

You now understand how my program provides you with the upper hand in controlling your destiny.

Later, I'll show you a method to help you determine, with close accuracy, the calories you need to eat to maintain your bodyweight. Without a laboratory measurement, we can't know precisely your TDEE. But,

Establishing the Basic Numbers

we can accomplish the most important goal which is to predict the total number of calories that you need to eat each day to maintain bodyweight.

The purpose behind these calculations is to help you understand that there are Laws in operation. These Laws determine your bodyweight. When you thoroughly understand the Laws, you'll be free of the bondage that has been created by the confusion foisted upon you by the misinformed, multi-billion dollar weight loss industry. These Laws are as inviolate as the fact that water freezes at 32 degrees.

What are the upper and lower limits of calorie burning in humans? Studies have measured the calorie burning at either extreme of physical activity: both at low-calorie outputs and at high-calorie outputs and provide a frame of reference for evaluating the results for the general population.

Non-ambulatory and chair-bound individuals expend the least amount of calories through physical activity each day. The TDEE from studies of these subjects was 1.21. This figure was slightly lower than the value of 1.27 suggested by the WHO as the survival requirement.

Maximum calorie burning over a limited time is different than the calorie burning that we can sustain over a long time. Maximum sustainable TDEE includes a Physical Activity Level that one follows as a way of life.

For example, the bicycle riders in the Tour de France had a TDEE (Total Daily Energy Expenditure) of 4.7 X RMR during the 21 days of the bicycle race. Other athletes involved in sled hauling across the Arctic achieved a TDEE of 4.5 during a 20-day event. In a study of male Nordic skiers, a TDEE value of 3.5 was the calorie burn of cross-country skiing. TDEEs of greater than 4.0 are above a level that's sustainable.

Studies of the calorie burns of athletes report that women burn between 2,700 and 4,300 calories a day. Men burn between 3,600-7,200 calories a day. This equals TDEEs of 2.0-3.5 X RMR and 2.5-4.0 X RMR. The highest TDEEs, 2.8 X RMR and 3.1 X RMR, were measured during periods of rigorous training. This level of calorie burning may be sustainable for limited periods of time but it's unlikely to represent the average for the whole year.

Lower TDEE values (2.0-2.3 X RMR) were recorded during periods of routine training suggesting that individuals can sustain this level of calorie burning for a long time.

Studies performed on soldiers indicate an energy output of 4,300 calories a day. This is a TDEE of 2.4 X RMR. Calorie burning for lumberjacks is 4,665 calories a day (TDEE = 2.6 X RMR). This indicates the heavy calorie requirements of that type of manual labor. This level of calorie burning is sustainable because these guys do it year after year as part of their employment.

The research data show that a TDEE range of 1.2-2.5 X RMR is sustainable. A TDEE of 2.5 X RMR indicates a heavy, physically active lifestyle. These ranges of TDEEs provide a rule-of-thumb guideline to the typical boundaries of sustainable physical activity levels. They indicate the usual calorie burning of the population.

●●●●●●●●●●●●●●●●●●●●●●●●●●●

In this last section I've covered the Total Daily Energy Expenditure (TDEE), a sum of your Resting Metabolic Rate (RMR) and your Physical Activity Level (PAL). As I've stated, RMR is the number of calories your body burns each day to maintain itself. You're obligated to burn this number of calories. The portion of calories that you burn above RMR is your PAL (Physical Activity Level). PAL is highly variable. It depends upon how much activity you do each day. A significant amount of scientific research supports the predictability of TDEE. This provides estimates for calculating an individual's daily calorie needs.

••••••••••••••••••••••••••••••

Accurate Determination of Total Daily Energy Expenditure (TDEE)

The technology to measure TDEE is available. But, this technology is both costly and not accessible for people. That's why so much research has gone into the development of other tools, such as the formulations I've outlined above so that people can accurately predict the number of calories they need to eat each day.

We can measure Resting Metabolic Rate (RMR) with a machine that measures the amount of oxygen consumed and the amount of carbon dioxide released. One is hooked up to the machine and he breathes into a hose for 30 minutes. We can measure TDEE by the doubly-labeled water technique. By subtracting RMR from TDEE, we determine one's physical activity level (PAL).

As a result of the studies completed over the last 20 years, we can accurately predict RMR (Resting Metabolic Rate) and Total Daily Energy Expenditure by using the mathematical formulas in this chapter.

Calculating Calorie Needs by Eating Food

There's another method for determining calorie needs, a method that is both accurate and inexpensive. This technique is called tritrimetry. This is like the technique we used to follow in chemistry class in the experiment in which one titrated a solution of acid with a base to reach neutrality. Do you remember this experiment from high school? Into a beaker of acid you slowly introduced single drops of base until you achieved a color change or a specific pH.

In the same way, we introduce measured amounts of calories into our body. We adjust the addition of calories until bodyweight remains stable. This way we reproduce our high school chemistry class technique of titration. This is a method to precisely determine daily calorie needs.

The procedure of tritrimetry follows: Buy a book listing the calorie content of different foods. Using the formulas I've provided, calculate both your RMR (Resting Metabolic Rate) and TDEE (Total Daily Energy Expenditure). Using the calculated number for TDEE as a starting point, eat that number of calories each day. Weigh yourself every day and record these values in a journal.

If the number of calories that you eat matches the number you're burning, your weight will remain stable. Obviously, there are some variations due to changes in water balance that affect bodyweight, therefore, you want to determine for at least one week, or two weeks, whether your weight remains stable to offset any weight changes because of water balance.

At the end of this first test, bodyweight will remain stable, decrease, or increase. If bodyweight decreases, the number of calories you're eating isn't adequate to meet your calorie needs. If bodyweight increases, the number of calories you're eating is more than you need.

We assume that a pound of fat has a calorie value of 3,500. (This notion, however, is extremely simplistic. I don't want to discuss the more complex matter here, now. I'll save that discussion for later chapters. In those chapters I'll provide you with the information to make the necessary adjustments. This complexity, however, in no way, invalidates this procedure.)

Now, if your weight didn't remain stable, calculate the number of calories you ate above or below the level necessary to sustain your desired bodyweight. Making minor adjustments to your daily calorie intake, you begin the procedure again. You repeat it until you've determined the precise number of calories needed in order to sustain your desired bodyweight.

For example, let's assume your calculated Total Daily Energy Expenditure (TDEE) is 2,500 calories a day. Using your book that lists the calories in foods, begin to consume 2,500 calories a day. At the end of one week, the scale shows that you've gained 1/2 pound. This is equivalent to an extra 1,750 calories intake above your calorie needs for the seven-day period.

Divide 1,750 by 7. This equals 250 calories a day. For the next week, make the adjustment by subtracting 250 calories from the 2,500 calories that you were eating. For the second week of your experiment, you'll eat 2,250 calories a day. Again, weigh yourself each day. At the end of the week, evaluate whether your weight has increased, decreased, or remained stable.

Does this seem like a lot of work? Its not, really. Obviously, the procedure of tritrimetry can be time-consuming. But, it's a perfect way to learn to obey the Laws. And, it's a perfect way to know exactly how many calories you need to eat each day.

This is the ultimate evaluation technique of my program. It's absolutely foolproof because it follows the Laws. It's a technique that I've used many times during my career to establish my own calorie needs. Once I was armed with this information, it became easy to determine the actions that I needed to take in order to become the master of my own body.

You can take this procedure to the limits. You do this by using liquid formulas making the control process of an exact calorie intake very easy. You can either purchase or make your own liquid diets. This process helps control the varied effects of different types of foods upon the water content of the body. I developed several recipes for drinks during my early years of attempting to understand the factors that control bodyweight.

In the market, today, there are many kinds of pre-packaged meals, drinks in a can, or powdered nutritional products. You can mix these with different types of liquids, including juices, water, or milk. All packaged foods now list the number of calories per serving. Therefore, it's easy to know exactly the number of calories you're consuming.

I'm an advocate of the low-carbohydrate diet. If you choose to follow that eating regimen, one of its significant features is that it causes diuresis (loss of water). This early water loss can be significant. And, water loss is one of the key features used by promoters of the low-carbohydrate diet to sell their program.

Be very clear about this, it's not fat loss; it's water loss. Therefore, if there's a significant loss of water weight, it'll be difficult, during the first few weeks, to use the technique of tritrimetry to establish your calorie needs. After several weeks of low-carbohydrate eating (or any diet), water balance returns to normal.

The primary benefit of low-carbohydrate eating is that the absence of carbohydrates suppresses appetite. It also induces changes in the body allowing some more fat tissue to be burned as energy. The low-carbohydrate diet slightly reduces the loss of LBM (Lean Body Mass),

Establishing the Basic Numbers

particularly muscle. In a later chapter, I'll describe fully all aspects of low-carbohydrate eating.

I encourage you, if you experiment with tritrimetry, to do it before switching to a low-carbohydrate diet. There's an important benefit in doing tritrimetry: during this initial phase of gaining control over your bodyweight, you'll establish baseline numbers that are specific to your own body.

If you start right off on a diet or exercise program, before establishing your baseline numbers, you'll likely see results from your program. But, now you've changed. And, since you didn't first acquire your basic numbers, you'll never know your baseline. Therefore, finding out where you are today serves as a foundation upon which you can base future decisions.

Find out where you are today, first, so you'll know where you are tomorrow.

The numbers are you, they're your history, and they're your future. Putting-it-to-the-numbers is, I believe, the most powerful weapon that you have in your arsenal against overweight and obesity. Our bodies operate under the Laws of Nature and it's foolhardy to try to escape from their power and it's also not possible.

The other **major obstacle** to the effective use of tritrimetry is that many overweight people mis-report the number of calories they eat each day. For this procedure to work, you must be brutally honest with yourself. You don't have to divulge these numbers to anyone other than yourself. So be honest and truthful. Your success depends upon it. If you discover that your calorie intake that maintains your bodyweight is well lower than predicted, you can be sure that you are kidding and deluding yourself about your calorie counting.

In short, the first phase of your program is to acquire

the information that serves as your road-map.

The calorie controls everything and nothing is more important than an understanding of the calorie.

Anything else that you do in your weight loss and weight control program is subordinate to the calorie. Programs *focusing* upon diet composition as the *primary* factor in helping you to lose weight are, simply, *wrong*.

There *are* benefits that you can achieve by changes in diet composition, particularly the low-carbohydrate diet, changes that make a significant contribution to the success of your program. But, they aren't the main factor.

Control of calories through the Energy Balance Equation *must* be your focal point.

●●●●●●●●●●●●●●●●●●●●●●●●●●●●

The preceding section provided information about a technique, tritrimetry, to guide you in determining the number of calories you need to eat each day to meet your energy needs. Tritrimetry is an inexpensive, yet precise, technique to establish your baseline, daily calorie needs.

●●●●●●●●●●●●●●●●●●●●●●●●●●●●

Two More Calculations

I'm already assuming that you've made an accurate determination of your bodyweight and your height. You had to in order to determine your RMR (Resting Metabolic Rate). The next calculation that you should make is that of your Body Mass Index (BMI). BMI is the standard measure used today to assess underweight, normal weight, overweight, and obesity. It's an important number that you should know.

Establishing the Basic Numbers

You can go onto my web site, (Chapter 4 Calculations www.ultimatedietsecrets.com), and have the program there do this calculation for you. If you want to do it on your own, now, here's the formula for calculating BMI:

Weight (kg) divided by height (meters squared) = Body Mass Index (BMI)

Also expressed as,

Wt (kg) ÷ Ht (m²) = Body Mass Index (BMI)

Weight in kilograms is pounds divided by 2.2. Calculate your height in meters squared by multiplying your height in inches by 2.54. Now, divide that by 100. Then square that number.

The ideal BMI (Body Mass Index) for both men and women is 21-22. The normal range is 18.5-24.9. Values below 18.5 are underweight and values greater than 24.9 are overweight. Values greater than 30.0 represent obesity.

BMI is a measure of the amount of weight you carry per unit height. BMI, however, doesn't tell you how much of your bodyweight is fat or lean tissue. A test to determine body composition is a much better barometer of your physical condition than BMI alone.

For example, the BMI of athletes, particularly those participating in power events, is often in the obese range because they have high amounts of muscle tissue. BMI is unable to differentiate muscle from fat.

Therefore, an accurate measure of body fat percent provides valuable information that contributes to your overall program. I've developed an accurate body composition program that provides a complete analysis of your body fat %, lean %, and body shape analysis. You can find the program on my companion web site, www.targetedbodysystems.com.

The program uses a measure of your body circumferences to calculate body fat %. Therefore, before going into the program at the site, have a tape measure available. The pages on the site provide a complete description of what and where to measure. After entering the measurements into the table, press the Go button. Within a few seconds the program provides your complete analysis.

The cost of the body composition analysis is only $9.95. You can periodically redo the test after beginning your weight loss program. It'll be very valuable to you to assess the changes you make. This is particularly true if you participate in another part of my program, my secret weapon: weight training. Weight training, of course, does more than any other activity to change the way you look.

● ●

Calculations of Body Mass Index and Body Composition are helpful in determining your present condition. This way, you can measure the effects created by your diet and/or exercise program. Of the two, Body Composition is a more precise measurement and provides the detailed information required to evaluate changes from diet and exercise.

● ●

Energy-In/Energy-Out

I've now described the fundamental Laws underpinning the regulation of bodyweight. I've also provided you with the means to determine your own calorie burn. Now, we can go on to a discussion of the factors that affect the Energy Balance Equation. The Energy Balance Equation comprises, as you now know,

Establishing the Basic Numbers

two sides: Energy-Out and Energy-In.

Anything that you do to control your weight **must** affect either one or both sides of the Equation. There is no other possibility.

RMR (Resting Metabolic Rate) is an "obligated function" of living. As a result, it's not amenable to change except under two conditions. As we've seen, it changes 1) in response to changes in the amount of calories consumed and 2) it changes in response to changes in bodyweight, particularly LBM (Lean Body Mass) with weight gain but not muscle gain. Later on, I'll discuss in more detail the adaptations in RMR to increases or decreases in both food intake and LBM.

Therefore, for the Energy-Out side of the Energy Balance Equation, we can only manipulate one part, the Physical Activity Level (PAL). We can't manipulate RMR and TEF (Thermic Effect of Food).

There are many ways to manipulate PAL. The primary ones include spontaneous physical activity and planned exercise activities.

For the Energy-In side of the Energy Balance Equation, our primary focus is on techniques to help control appetite. This is the biological drive to eat. It's extremely important to understand that appetite is programmed into each and every cell.

The consumption of foods to acquire energy (calories) is an essential feature of living organisms. Without fuel, life isn't possible.

Biological drives are virtually impossible to overcome by **Willpower**. This is one of the major pitfalls in most weight loss and weight control programs. These programs demand that the individual demonstrate remarkable Willpower to succeed. It's my contention that Willpower never overcomes a Biological drive.

Our focus in detailing the Energy-In portion of the Energy Balance Equation is on methods to control appetite. Physical activity and diet composition have a very powerful influence upon appetite.

Remember, appetite is not something solely of the mind. It's a function of many signals released by individual cells requesting food. These cells are collective members of individual organs. The organs are themselves collective members of the whole body.

The organization of complex organisms is such that an individual cell can't provide for its own needs. As a result, each cell is now dependent on other cells, organs, and systems to provide its requirements for life. Systems have evolved within the body to protect the cell and maintain life. There's an extraordinary amount of interdependency among the parts of the system. The messages and the communication networks of the human body make the Internet seem like the creation of a precocious child.

● ●

At this juncture, I've established the legitimacy of the Energy Balance Equation and its two sides, Energy-In and Energy-Out.

The focus of the remaining portions of this book is upon dissecting each of these two sides. I'll develop effective protocols that you can use to make desired changes in your body.

Additionally, I've shown that the preponderance of scientific research convincingly demonstrates that there's no evidence of a genetic or metabolic defect responsible for obesity. Therefore, we don't need to spend any more time thinking that there's something wrong with our glands. Or our genes either.

There is, clearly, variation in the calorie needs of seemingly similar subjects. But the reasons underlying these differences are readily evaluated with the techniques that I've outlined above.

Obesity only develops, however, if an individual fails to match his calorie intake to his calorie needs.

I can state, unequivocally, that the primary cause of obesity is an individual's inability to match calorie intake with calorie output.

Obesity is, therefore, ultimately determined by the behavior of man in the modern world. It's a maladaptation to behavioral and environmental pressures, a maladaptation that drives people to consume more food than they need. And, it pushes them to move less. Thus, modern-life has led to a significant decrease in daily calorie burn.

Interestingly though, recent research has indicated that calorie intake has actually decreased over the last several decades. Yet obesity continues to climb. So, even the availability of tasty and abundant foods doesn't appear to be the primary problem in the cause of obesity.

The only conclusion that we can venture is that calorie burning has decreased more than food intake has decreased.

The Second Law of Thermodynamics is one of the few incontrovertible facts in nutrition. So, food intake has decreased and we're still getting fatter. Something, therefore, must have happened to the Energy-Out side of the Energy Balance Equation.

And, that's exactly what's happened, as I've just said. People are decreasing their calorie burning by decreasing their physical activity.

In summary, I've established the basic facts responsible for the control and maintenance of bodyweight. Now, I'll discuss at length the choices that you can make to allow Nature to work more effectively on your behalf.

Things are really getting exciting now. As you can see, we're resolving many of the unexplained and confusing factors involved in the control of bodyweight and setting a level of priority to all of the factors involved.

Your Power to Control is rapidly increasing.

Chapter 4

Growing Up in the Fitness Revolution

Let's take a look at what I encountered in my effort to solve my obesity problem. The dietary regimens most often promulgated by those in the physical culture movement (a movement I was thrust into because of my interest in muscle building) were, during my early years, oriented toward vegetarianism. This included an emphasis on whole, live foods: fruits, vegetables, and grains, ideas so very popular today. Further, the New Age movement, arising in the late 1960's, and booming by the early 1970's, spawned many books and articles that preached that the ideal diet for humans was grain/vegetable/fruit-based. People in the diet-based health movement made recommendations that contrasted to those in the hard-core bodybuilding community that pre-dated the steroid era.

Although my first attempts to lose weight were effective, they hadn't led to any long-term nutritional knowledge or benefits. In my late teenage years, I'd acquired no real knowledge about the effects of manipulating calories or how to use the diet composition tool to improve my results. Diet composition is about the protein, carbohydrate, and fat content of the diet. I did, however, come to realize that I needed to effect a reduction in my total calorie intake. I want to present some of my actual experiments so you can see what I went through to learn all about bodyweight regulation.

Adelle Davis's book, <u>Let's Eat Right to Keep Fit</u>, provided the solution: a formula diet she'd concocted and named "Pep-Up." One of the chapters in her book was titled, "Health and Normal Weight Go Hand in Hand." In this chapter she laid out her ideas about reducing body fat. Pep-Up seemed the perfect solution to my over-fat condition. Pep-Up would allow me to perfectly control my calorie intake. This reduced the chance of inadvertently consuming more food than desired.

I prepared several pages of paper and listed the ingredients in the formula. Then I determined the calorie content, along with the grams of protein in the total day's volume of fluid. Below is the formula copied from my notes made in 1972.

Food Item	**Calories**	**Protein (gr.)**
2 tbsp. lecithin	105	0
2 eggs	150	12
2 tbsp. oil	250	0
¼ cup yogurt	30	2
1 cup skim milk powder	434	45
¼ cup protein powder	103	18
¼ cup yeast powder	150	20
¼ cup de-fatted soy flour	115	10
¼ cup wheat germ	60	4
3 oz. orange juice	165	0
1½ tsp. calcium lactate powder		
½ tsp. magnesium oxide powder		
1 tsp. vanilla		
Water		
	1,562 calories	111 protein grams

Dr. Gregory Ellis's Ultimate Diet Secrets Lite

I placed all of the ingredients into a blender, using enough water to bring the volume of the drink to one quart. After mixing, I poured the blended ingredients into my two-quart, stainless steel Stanley thermos. I supplemented the drink with kelp tablets and liver tablets.

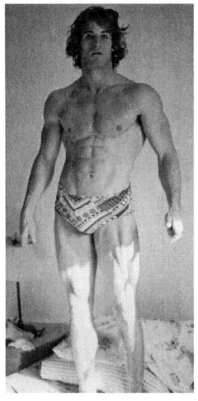

After first Pep-Up, Thanksgiving 1972, bodyweight at 187 pounds with well-defined abdominals.

Every three hours, I would un-cap the Stanley thermos and take three, equally mouth-filling swigs of fluid. You can imagine, from studying the ingredients in the table, above, that the taste was absolutely disgusting. Worse yet, is the fact that the ingredients would settle deeply within the minuscule crevices in my tongue. They remained there, scorching my taste buds for at least the next hour. No amount of swishing with water seemed to dislodge these well-entrenched particles from my tongue.

This weight loss experiment was a perfectly calorie-controlled regimen. So, the only additional thing that I could put in my mouth each day was water.

Eager to begin my weight loss program, I began consuming my Pep-Up formula on September 22, 1972. My starting bodyweight was 218 pounds. I took three swigs, every three hours, six times a day, from then until November 23, 1972. Not only was I famished, I suffered because of the boredom and the lack of chewing. The only reward was the rate at which fat peeled from my body. In addition to the exactness with which I controlled my daily intake of calories, I began to record my bodyweight each day. This is a practice I still continue today. After the first week I'd reduced my bodyweight by 5½ pounds. This was a loss consistent with the proclamations of the quick weight loss hucksters, still with us today. The second week's weight loss slowed, only 3½ pounds. This rate of loss continued throughout the duration of my program. I ended the Pep-Up regimen at Thanksgiving. The concoction helped me to reduce my weight to 187 pounds. This was the leanest I'd ever been in my life; I sported a well-defined set of abdominal muscles. My body was essentially devoid of extraneous fat. I'd attained my immediate goal of diet success. And at the same time, I achieved a long-standing dream, first imagined when I was twelve years old.

I was ecstatic over my success, knowing now that I could do it and that I had done it. What I didn't realize is that I had only scratched the surface of my understanding of weight loss and weight control. The future held many more surprises.

I had no understanding, then, of the ironclad Laws that I've already described to you. I did what you're supposed to do on a Thanksgiving holiday and feasted that Thanksgiving Day, the 23rd of November 1972. I made up for all my suffering of the preceding two months. Already, by the day after Thanksgiving, I'd regained weight. The scale groaned under my six pounds of "new" flesh; I weighed 193 pounds.

● ●

My over-consumption of food didn't stop at the end of Thanksgiving. And I immediately returned to my pre-diet pattern of eating. By November 30th, I'd gained another 5 pounds, tipping the scale at 198. I remained relatively stable at that weight throughout December. Then, on the day after Christmas I reached 202 pounds. I now had a net gain of 15 pounds since the end of my diet. The weight gain continued throughout January. I reached 210 pounds by February 4th, 213 pounds by February 19th, 217 pounds by March 8th, and 226 pounds by April 17th.

I regained all the weight I'd lost. Even worse, I'd overshot my previous high weight by an additional eight pounds. Obviously, my abdominal muscles were gone, disappearing long before I'd reached 226 pounds. They were gone by the time I'd reached 208 pounds. I was disgusted with my weight gain and the disappearance of my muscular definition. Something had to be done. So, on April 23rd I began yet another diet using the Pep-Up formulation. I was a glutton for punishment. Again, as before, the weight disappeared rapidly. I dropped 6 pounds the first week, 4 more during the second week, 3 pounds in the third week, and so on. Finally, I reached a weight of 195 pounds on June 8th. After this weight loss, again, I regained, climbing to 200 pounds. I maintained that weight throughout the summer until late August when I began to experience increasing weight to about 207-208 pounds. In October, I began another diet at a starting weight of 208 pounds. This time I reduced myself to 185 pounds by Thanksgiving of 1973. This was right back to about the weight that I'd attained a year earlier.

I was, however, slowly learning something about weight control: nothing, yet, implanted in my consciousness, but the sense that one had to consume less food in order to sustain a lower bodyweight: nothing that I could put numbers on despite all the success I'd experienced on the rigorously controlled Pep-Up formulation. The only time that I'd paid attention to my calorie intake was while I was on Pep-Up. The moment I came off the drink, I ate whatever I wanted. This is just as most people do when ending a weight loss period.

I began gradually, almost by instinct, to reduce the amount of food that I consumed. There was nothing, at this time, systematic about the process. Obviously, this "instinctual" method was not very reliable. I was still many years away from making the necessary connections that would allow me to avoid these wild swings in bodyweight. It would take years before I developed patterns of behavior that would allow me to attain and maintain my goals.

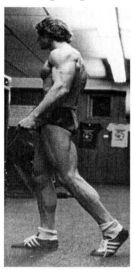
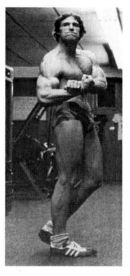

Two photos after using the 800-calorie Pep-Up drink and stripping off most of my body fat. January 1974, bodyweight 178 pounds.

My weight fluctuations were extraordinarily wide. This was a function of my limited understanding of the methods necessary to lose weight and to the control of my eating patterns. I continued to study exercise, nutritional supplementation, and food intake as they related to health improvement. Unfortunately, I was confounding all of my experiments by trying to accomplish multiple tasks, simultaneously. This led to confusion: the inability to separate the results of one experiment from the other.

This became all the more confusing as a function of my decision to become a vegetarian. I was influenced to make this decision by the health writers of the day. They espoused the many health benefits that were supposedly associated with vegetarianism.

I was narrowing, gradually, the wide swings in weight change, beginning each new diet at a lower bodyweight. There was now a critical difference. I now knew the bodyweight I needed to attain to be free of body fat. At least that part of my long journey was now over. This provided the essential frame of reference against which I could measure all of my future experiments. When 1973 ended, I had consistently maintained my weight between 188-195 pounds. By January 5, 1974, I'd reached 200 pounds. This weight was about 15 pounds heavier than my well-established "little-fat-on-the-body" ideal weight.

At that juncture, I chose to begin another diet before things got out of hand again. I returned to the Pep-Up formula with which I'd had so much success. But this time there was a major modification: I reduced the quantity of the ingredients by exactly one-half. This cut my daily calorie intake to 800. This was difficult, but I stayed on this diet through the end of January. I reached 178 pounds, a record low bodyweight for me. Again, the end of the diet led to an increased consumption of food, increasing my weight to 189 pounds by February 7th. Throughout the winter and spring, my weight continued to climb, reaching 205 pounds by early May. Here was, again, a repetition of the consistent pattern of yo-yoing weight loss and weight regain. Even my commitment to vegetarianism didn't prevent my continued accumulation of weight (and fat).

Growing Up in the Fitness Revolution

● ●

I began to wean myself from the Pep-Up formula because of the severe challenge of this strict, hard-to-do regimen. Throughout this period of time, whenever I hit a bodyweight of about 210 pounds, I'd institute another bout of dieting. My weight charts are riddled with the phrases "Began Diet" and "End Diet." I was finding it more and more difficult to maintain these strict reducing periods long enough to attain my 185-pound ideal.

The only available arbiters were my scale, my eyes, and a tape measure.

My body goals were always two-fold (three-fold, if you count my interest in eating for good health). The goals were to maximize muscle mass while minimizing fat mass. During 1973-1975, I had not yet availed myself of sophisticated measuring devices. I allowed my reason and observations to dictate my understanding of the results of my various experiments.

It's through hindsight, now, that I can state, unequivocally, that I constantly deluded myself. I ignored what my eyes actually told me, believing what I wanted to believe. Like the obese subject, convinced that he's not eating much, I had complete confidence in the interpretations I made. Anytime that I began a new training or diet program, I convinced myself that I was adding muscle at a fast rate. In this view, then, I believed that my weight gain was all muscle. I told myself that the weight gain couldn't be fat, had to be muscle, a mistake that I consistently made throughout many decades, even as recently as 1998. (I do believe, however, that that was the last time I'll make this mistake.)

I continued my weight loss/weight gain process regularly throughout the rest of 1974, 1975, and into the early part of 1976. Sometimes my diets would be more successful than others, bringing me to a bodyweight of about 180 pounds. The upper limit of my weight "regain" seemed to top-out, usually, at about 210-215 pounds. I was thoroughly ensconced in my vegetarian lifestyle. I berated anyone who failed to agree with my viewpoint. I vilified meat eaters, damning them for their sins against God, society, and the environment.

A natural extension of the vegetarian movement, with its emphasis on maintaining a clean colon, was a belief in the value of fasting. The growing interest in health created an ocean of writers who preached the positive aspects of regular fasting. This, of course, piqued my interest, particularly because it suited my extreme nature.

Although I'd attained a high degree of muscular definition, I'd been unable to sustain it. When I gained weight, I hated to lose my defined appearance. I was perplexed at my failure to maintain it.

Because of this frustration, I planned a new

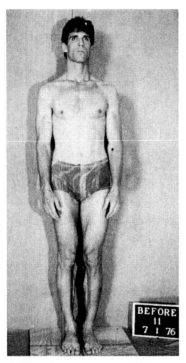

After reducing body fat to a low level, the body rapidly eats its muscles. This is what happened during my fasting experiments when I completely stripped myself of <u>both</u> fat and muscle.

extreme regimen, my most extreme ever. In April 1976, I undertook a self-imposed fast. I allowed myself nothing more than 2 oz. of fruit juice each day. Juice was the elixir of the Gods, my books informed me. My daily juice intake was well under 80 calories. I started the fast weighing 194 pounds. I drank my "glass" of juice in sips throughout the day. The fast continued for nine days. I reached a final, end-of-diet bodyweight of 176 pounds.

A rapid regain, of course, followed and pushed my weight, over the ensuing 25 days, to 185 pounds.

The amount of leanness that I achieved was remarkable. I was, however, unaware about how much I was actually shrinking, not only in body fat, but also in muscle as well. I didn't want to face the fact that I was also losing my hard-earned muscles. Although my muscles shriveled, the muscle that remained stood out in bold relief. This was a look that I'd desired from the time I was 12-years-old. I'd become so obsessed with my appearance, in fact, that even a weight regain to 183 pounds was more than I could bear. As a result, I embarked upon another 12-day fast. With this one I reduced my weight to 164.5 pounds.

Amazingly, this was 100 pounds less than the weight I'd achieved in my several-years-earlier bulking-up phase.

Again, as always, I immediately rebounded: my weight increased by 13 pounds over the next 17 days. Reaching 180 pounds again, I instituted another fast, reducing my weight to 174 pounds, thereafter rebounding almost immediately to 186 pounds.

Ever so slowly, though, I was beginning to learn that I couldn't consume much food if I wanted to maintain the lower bodyweight. And that's exactly what I did: ate sparingly. I also began to employ other so-called "health" regimens promulgated by the vegetarian cultists. This included the regular use of two-quart coffee enemas, the eating of wheat sprouts, olive oil liver flushes, raw foods, and food combining. I followed Dr. Arnold Ehret's Mucousless Diet Healing System.

As my extremeness expanded, I came to believe that, if one became spiritual enough, he could live on no food at all. He could subsist solely on breath. I never made it that far. Fortunately, I began, gradually, to move away from these other "health" practices. Surprisingly, many of them, here in the year 2002, have become commonplace, practiced by many otherwise sane people.

The fast had been extremely difficult. I don't believe that anything that I ever did in my life was as difficult as these fasts, repeated back-to-back. It was even harder then some of my most grueling workouts.

I became so exhausted from these fasts that it was difficult to perform the most menial tasks.

The second fast, reducing my bodyweight to 165 pounds, occurred in late June/early July, a time of rising summer temperatures. I remember lying in bed one morning, covered only by a single sheet. It was too warm for anything more. I remember wanting to turn over. But, I found it almost impossible to overcome the weight of the sheet. Anytime I stood up, either from lying down or rising from a chair, I almost blacked out. I later found out that this condition, postural hypotension, resulted from the inability of my body to adjust to the rapid change in posture by providing enough blood flow to my brain. This meant that my nervous system, my circulatory system, and my hormonal system were severely compromised as a result of my fast (starvation).

I continued, on and off, with more fasting and other, less rigorous, weight loss attempts. Indeed, my weight record charts are punctuated with unceasing attempts to attain the lean, well-chiseled look that I desired. It seemed, to me, that I'd begun to throttle back on the very wide fluctuations in weight loss/regain. I had begun to achieve more stability, maintaining myself in the 180-190 pound range. I was, at this point, able to make sophisticated scientific evaluations as a result of my graduate programs.

I began to understand the idea of body composition, the fractionation of bodyweight into its two primary components -- fat tissue and lean tissue.

The gold standard in the determination of body composition is a technique called underwater weighing, based on Archimedes' principles. On June 27, 1977, I was immersed, for the first time, in a tank of warm water to have my underwater weight measured. Plugging his weight into a mathematical formula, one can accurately calculate his body fat percent. I weighed 181 pounds that day, and my calculated body fat was 5.7%, astonishingly low.

I now, finally, had confirmation of what my eyes had been telling me: I was lean, very lean. I also was becoming successful at maintaining this low bodyweight and body fat percent. I was still a vegetarian throughout this period, consuming painfully small amounts of food each day. Again, in 1978, I immersed myself in the tank of water, and my calculated body fat was 5.36%. Although I was maintaining weight stability, it was difficult. It required the consumption of far less food than I actually wanted to eat. I came to be aware, but not fully conscious, of the difference between the amount of food that I could consume at a bodyweight of 175-185 and the amount I could consume at a bodyweight of 220-225. This awareness came, later, to be a fully-flowered conscious knowledge. It's an important concept and I'll discuss it in detail later.

I didn't realize at that time how rigorously and scientifically I'd designed my personal experiments. Even today, there are few scientific studies exploring the responses to the extreme reduction in calories that I underwent in my experiments. Further, there isn't much literature that explores the results accruing to experiments in extensive overfeeding. This is the technique that I used in my bulking-up phase, leading to my peak bodyweight of 265 pounds. Researchers, in the 1960's, had only begun to explore the physical changes that result from overfeeding. Therefore, there was very little information, in those early years, that was available to me about the changes that I was experiencing during my cutting-edge experiments.

Chapter 5

Learning How to Take Control of My Body

My experience and knowledge increased because of my personal experiments. And now, as a graduate student in a medical school physiology department, I was also immersing myself into the teachings of scientists engaged in the study of weight loss methods. Most often these experiments were conducted by medical doctors who are not scientists. The experiments do reach an outcome by the following of a particular dietary scheme but do little to teach any of the underlying biochemical or physiological facts involved in what happens to a body undergoing a weight loss program. Nonetheless, these studies do make some contribution to our understanding.

Medical doctors studying weight control during the late 1970's and early 1980's came up with a development for weight loss called the Very Low Calorie Diet (VLCD). It became very popular, spawning several commercial companies that manufactured the pouch-powder used as the day's calorie intake. These companies promoted the diet as the answer to an ever-increasing national obesity epidemic.

The value of this dietary treatment was the rapid weight loss that occurred. The major difficulty, however, with the VLCD was that it significantly depressed the Resting Metabolic Rate (RMR). It caused a large loss of LBM (Lean Body Mass: muscle tissue and organs). These two changes were always cataclysmic to weight loss and weight control success.

Researchers tried diligently and relentlessly to develop methods to minimize the impact of the VLCD on these two parameters. The calorie content of the VLCD ranged between 400-600 calories a day. One technique the theorists posited in order to minimize the decline in RMR and LBM was to provide the majority of the calories as protein. As a result, much scientific research was directed toward this end.

I had another idea about preserving RMR and LBM. I began to work with researchers at the renowned University of Pennsylvania Obesity Research Group, in Philadelphia. I proposed that we implement a weight training program in an effort to minimize the loss of muscle tissue, a novel idea at that time. I wanted to compare weight training with endurance exercise, and then compare both to a non-exercise control group. We decided to test my hypothesis in rats. Workers at Thomas Jefferson University, in Philadelphia, had developed a strength training protocol for rats. They'd place a harness over the rat's back that had slots for adding weights. They'd add ever-increasing amounts of weight while stimulating the rat to climb an inclined ladder repeatedly. After the experimental period, I was going to terminate the animals, homogenize them in a blender, and determine each one's body composition: the proportions of water, protein, and fat.

Researchers at Columbia University, in New York City, had the necessary expertise to teach me these techniques of body composition analysis. No one in the Philadelphia institutions did. One of the New York researchers was to serve as my co-thesis advisor. In addition to the body composition analysis, she wanted me to measure the animal's oxygen use (to determine the calorie burn) during a graded exercise test. This was an extraordinarily cumbersome and highly technical measurement, a Ph. D. dissertation research project on its own. Unable to talk any sense into her about abandoning this idea, I had to scrap this project.

This was, however, the beginning of my intensive study into body composition.

The vast majority of people who undertake a weight loss and weight control program are only concerned about the amount of **weight** they lose. This is a critical mistake and should never be the focus of their efforts to change their appearance. The goal of the program should always be to lose the most amount of **fat** possible. At the same time, one should focus on either minimizing the loss of Lean Body Mass, maintaining Lean Body Mass, or increasing the amount of Lean Body Mass, in the form of **muscle**.

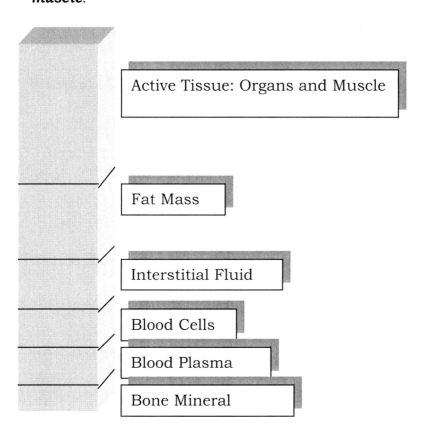

Learning How to Take Control of My Body

The largest two components of body composition, the ones with which we are most concerned, are the two tissues: the Lean Body Mass, composed of muscle tissue and organs, and the adipose tissue or Fat Mass. As a result of my studies into body composition, my focus shifted from absolute weight loss to uncovering effective techniques to reduce body fat. At the same time, the program must preserve or increase Lean Body Mass, particularly muscle since it is difficult to achieve any voluntary control over organ size. Although I understood the idea of changing the individual components, I had not, as yet, begun the study of potential methods to influence changes specifically in the separate components. I, like most people, had focused upon absolute losses in bodyweight. But I'd been fortunate in discovering weight training during the formulation of my own programs. Weight training was, and is, the most effective method to maintain or increase muscle tissue. I'd been lucky to stumble into it as a youngster.

In 1977, soon after I completed the medical school biochemistry course, I began studying how the body regulates its metabolism. This is a complicated subject filled with minute details. My studies required the mastery of a wide range of individual subjects. I dreaded the amount of work that I knew was required to master the regulation of metabolism. It was to be an arduous task. I knew, though, that an understanding of these mechanisms was critical to unraveling the secrets behind losing fat and building muscle.

The body regulates its metabolism primarily through enzymes. Enzymes are the stuff of life. Signals coming from the nervous system and the hormonal system tell the cellular enzymes what to do in response to an ever-changing environment. There was no question in my mind that I had to have a thorough understanding of the factors affecting changes in enzymes. This included all factors that affect enzyme **levels** and **activity**. Changes at the cellular level were at the heart of how to control the muscle and Fat Mass at the whole body level.

The two primary fuels used to power muscular contraction are glucose (sugar) and fat. My research into metabolic regulation had provided me with a preliminary understanding of fuel use. I understood about the determinants of how the body regulates the use of these two fuels, fat and carbohydrate.

●●●●●●●●●●●●●●●●●●●●●●●●●●●

During these years, I continued to vary my own training programs, experimenting with different weightlifting programs. I also used other activities such as cardiovascular conditioning through running or bicycling. These programs of training were always coordinated with some form of dietary manipulation in my unceasing attempts to find the most effective methods. I was trying to refine my understanding of how to manipulate and mold my body. My early, extreme, methods were, obviously, not the answer. They did, however, provide the necessary first steps toward making further refinements.

Unfortunately, although I had been highly trained academically by this time, I was still subject to the promises about miracles in fat loss and muscle building presented in the popular magazines. These programs were promulgated by many of the highly-publicized "experts" who were always popping-up on the national scene. In my mind, I hadn't yet become a "they" of the "they say" group. I still followed instead of leading.

By the mid-1980's, the complex carbohydrate diet became the dietary darling of both health enhancement and performance enhancement. Fat was ridiculed. Many myths began to surround the movement that supported the use of complex carbohydrates and the eschewal of fat with all its perceived dangers.

I was also drawn into this movement because I was still several years away from understanding the mechanisms, and the misinformation, surrounding the metabolism of complex carbohydrates and fats in man and animals.

My daily weight charts demonstrate that I continued to experiment with periods of weight loss. I continued my efforts to discover optimal programs for attaining my goal of maximizing fat loss and either maintaining or increasing muscle tissue. I continued to fluctuate between the same range of bodyweights that appeared to be my upper limit (220 pounds) and lower limit (190 pounds). My notes also indicate that I'd begun to employ calorie counting as a method of weight and body composition control. It was, though, not yet my focal point.

I built my own research center and now I could conduct a very detailed analysis of the results of my varied training and dietary regimens. Periodically, after several months of a new experimental training/diet program, I would immerse myself into the tank of water. I would calculate my Fat Mass and Lean Body Mass to assess the changes occurring from the regimen. The surprising finding, that continued to repeat itself, was that any new weight gain, or weight loss, was always, consistently, the same. Whenever I gained weight, 75% of the gain was Fat Mass and 25% was Lean Body Mass. Conversely, any weight loss was represented by a loss of 75% fat and 25% lean. I was always amazed by the continuity of these accurately measured changes. This is because I'd convinced myself that the weight gain I'd achieved was mostly lean (muscle). This, obviously, helped me to achieve a more discerning eye relative to future changes in my clients or me.

As a result of these consistent changes, I was now able to reject the complex carbohydrate dietary regimen. It possessed no magical powers to increase muscle and decrease fat. I began to think that I'd reached my genetic limits and that further change might not be possible.

••••••••••••••••••••••••••••

I took the medical school biochemistry course in 1977. It was in this course that I'd learned the basic metabolic pathways involved in the breakdown of food into a source of fuel for the body. In the following years, I'd taken it upon myself to delve more deeply into the study of metabolic pathways. I became particularly interested in the **control mechanisms** determining the flow of fuels between different tissues. Obviously, I was looking for any information that would guide me in the selection of methods for increasing muscle mass while, at the same time, decreasing fat. To complete my Ph. D. dissertation, I had to dig as deeply as I possibly could into enzymes, metabolic pathways, and metabolic regulation. I had to understand the mechanisms relating to carbohydrate metabolism. I also, however, had to understand all aspects of fat metabolism. And most important, I had to understand the **interrelationship** between fat and carbohydrate metabolism.

As it turned out, I couldn't have selected a better project for my dissertation than the one I chose because this research provided me with both a Ph. D. degree and an intimate understanding of the use of food as fuel. I understood how the body processed food as fuel all the way down to the genes that coded for manufacturing the enzymes responsible for controlling fuel use.

I also gained a completely new appreciation of fat. Since I'd come to understand that fat was not the cause of coronary heart disease, I felt safe in exploring its many dietary and nutritional benefits. It's a marvelous tissue.

So, I began to explore the idea of increasing my own consumption of fat, a truly heretical decision.

It wasn't until 1960 that researchers determined the purpose of the fat that for years they'd seen circulating in the bloodstream. During the next decade, a vast body of scientific literature grew at a dizzying pace and uncovered many details about the way the body processes fat as fuel.

One of my most interesting discoveries was that fat was proven as the preferred source of fuel by the body's tissues. This idea was in direct conflict with the majority who, here in 2003, still believe that glucose (blood sugar) and its storage form, glycogen, are the primary sources of fuel that power the body's metabolic processes.

The **critical** feature of the high-fat diet, however, was that one had to follow the diet for at least several weeks. This was the only way one could realize the improved work output provided by the high-fat intake.

This, of course, was in direct conflict with the many hundreds of studies supporting the use of high-carbohydrate diets, and particularly the technique of glycogen loading, to enhance endurance. I cannot dispute the veracity of the glycogen loading experiments; they've been reproduced in so many laboratories that the results are indisputable.

These studies, however, were always performed under the constraints of a seven-day experimental period. No one ever extended the studies beyond one week. When such extended studies were finally tried, it was discovered that the body needed several weeks, at least, to adapt itself to the use of fat as the primary source of fuel. It takes about one month for the body to manufacture enough of the enzymes that are necessary to efficiently break down fat into smaller molecules. From these smaller molecules the cells extract the energy to perform work via their new "fat-breaking-down" and "fat-burning enzymes."

This metabolic adaptation takes time to occur. In the absence of a high-fat intake, the body automatically breaks down and reduces the amount of the enzymes that are responsible for fat metabolism because it's wasteful to the body-machine to maintain them. Conversely, in the presence of a high-carbohydrate intake, the body manufactures the enzymes necessary to break down carbohydrates. Researchers didn't understand this metabolic economy. As a result, they failed to set up the appropriate experiments to uncover the importance of fat as a source of fuel for body tissues.

Sadly, the researchers who discovered that a high-fat intake led to increased endurance -- beyond that which could be provided by carbohydrates -- would not condone the use of a high-fat diet. Why? This answer is simple: they also had been snowed by the phony scientific literature implicating fat as the cause of heart disease. They never questioned these ideas, accepting what they had "learned," heard, from the Establishment. The result, today, is that little research is performed exploring fat as a source of fuel because of the erroneous belief that increasing one's fat intake is dangerous.

● ●

My studies had armed me with a detailed understanding of the biochemistry and the regulation of metabolism. I'd become so enamored with fat that it was very easy for me to make the next step toward a major change in my diet. I was aware of the low-carbohydrate diet, particularly the Atkins version. I hadn't yet used a low-carbohydrate diet as part of my regimen, or so I thought.

Learning How to Take Control of My Body

Looking back at my earliest bodybuilding years, though, I realized that I had fallen into a low-carbohydrate diet at that time almost instinctively. I consumed, in those years, enormous quantities of protein powder and meats.

I decided to begin the Atkins version of the low-carbohydrate diet. Within one week I gained 5 pounds, an unexpected result based on Atkins' promises and proclamations. The key feature promoted by the Atkins version of the low-carbohydrate diet is to eat as much food as you want as long as you reduce carbohydrates. **Atkins is absolutely convinced that calories aren't involved in the control of bodyweight -- he states that strongly and repeatedly in his writings.** In the very first week of my Atkins trial, I discovered how wrong he was.

I moved towards the Atkins regimen because it was the most visible exposition about low-carbohydrate eating. At that time, however, I was still several years away from understanding the overarching control exerted by the Energy Balance Equation (calories in vs. calories out). Therefore, I blindly followed Atkins' idea that calories don't matter. The result: I gained five pounds in the process!

After that experience, I embarked upon my own study of diet composition (coming to perceive of myself as "they" in the phrase "they say"). My focus was on uncovering exactly where Atkins had gone wrong. I knew it had to do with calories, but didn't yet see precisely how he had fallen into his error of observation. (I found out later and, in my writing, I tell you all about this major mistake *in*, and limitation *to*, Atkins' diet plan. It's a downloadable piece from my web site order page.)

Chapter 6

How Weight Loss (and Gain) Affect Body Composition

The parts of body composition and the chemical processes of life are highly regulated. They're automatically controlled.

And for most body parts, the processes controlling them **aren't** under voluntary control. We can make voluntary choices that adjust these controls, but we can't change them.

People are always saying how different every one is. What works for one person, they say, won't work for another. I agree that there's variability among different people. However, I disagree with the idea that the variability is extreme. In other words, one's legs may be longer or shorter, thicker or thinner than another's. But, nonetheless, we all have only two legs, not three or four.

This is also true for our body composition: we are all made up of exactly the same basic stuff.

And there are control mechanisms that regulate the amount of each element (the stuff). These control mechanisms maintain precise, healthy levels of this stuff. Some elements are tightly regulated, hardly deviating from the average value. This includes elements such as blood levels of sodium and potassium. If these elements deviate from their narrow, normal ranges, there's a threat to life itself.

Bodyweight is also a precisely regulated process. It varies, though, within wider ranges. Here, wider variations are more easily tolerated and there's less threat to life such as would occur if one's blood sugar

How Weight Loss (and Gain) Affect Body Composition

values varied over as wide a range. (Of course, this occurs in diseases such as diabetes, a life-threatening condition.)

We've made startling advances during the last two decades in measuring calorie balance. Our studies have provided researchers with a detailed understanding about the genetic and metabolic basis of obesity.

In the overwhelming majority of cases, there isn't any evidence of a **genetic** or **metabolic** defect responsible for obesity. Our detailed understanding of the body's in-born capacity to self-regulate bodyweight shows that the causes of overweight arise because of **behavioral** and **environmental** factors. These behavioral and environmental factors include overeating and too little physical activity. Later, I'll develop my thesis that the **primary** cause of overweight and obesity is a too-low level of physical activity.

Data from the United Kingdom show that since 1970 food intake has decreased. Yet, simultaneously, an increase in bodyweight occurred. The paradox of increasing obesity, at a time of decreasing food consumption, has only one explanation. This is that there has been an even more profound decrease in calorie burning. This unbalances the Energy Balance Equation toward increased bodyweight.

As I've stated, <u>ad nauseam</u>, overweight and obesity develop only if one fails to match his calorie burn to his calorie intake.

Therefore, the primary factor in overweight and obesity lies in the failure to match calorie burning to calorie intake.

Throughout this book, I'll continue to develop this fact. I'll also show you how to use strategies to fine tune each side of the Energy Balance Equation. With this information in hand, you'll derive more "bang-for-your-buck" from its use.

I've now established that bodyweight is highly regulated. All aspects of this precise regulation are subject to my thesis in weight loss and weight control: "putting-it-to-the-numbers," a method of seeing if broad based statements make any sense in reality.

In this section, I'll describe the **predictable** changes that occur in body composition with bodyweight loss or gain. These changes arise from **any** diet program. This is because all methods to lose bodyweight are subject to the Laws I've described.

We need to consider only two parts of body composition for our discussion. These are the **Fat Mass** (adipose tissue) and **Lean Body Mass** (organs and muscle).

Let's look at what happens when people lose bodyweight. The criterion for most people in evaluating the "success" of their weight loss program is the amount, in pounds, of weight that is lost. They don't consider its composition, **Fat Mass** or **Lean Body Mass**.

But what people really should lose is fat, not Lean Body Mass, muscles and organs. Most people, however, just don't know that this is the correct goal. That's because no one has ever taught them the facts about bodyweight loss, until now. No one has ever helped them refine their weight loss practice.

Adults exhibit individual variability in their body composition (Lean Body Mass and Fat Mass content). This is the same as the variations they experience in height and weight, and in other body functions such as RMR (Resting Metabolic Rate) and muscle strength. I must emphasize, however, that the variability in Lean Body Mass is much less than that for Fat Mass.

How Weight Loss (and Gain) Affect Body Composition

As a result, large variations in bodyweight are usually accounted for by large variations in Fat Mass. The body's controls to limit wide variations in Lean Body Mass do not operate in Fat Mass losses or gains.

The blood, for example, can vary only within narrow limits. In contrast, though, the wide range of variation in the amount of muscle and fat that is compatible with health and life is truly amazing.

There's a vast amount of scientific literature describing the changes in bodyweight and its composition in people who diet or exercise. These research studies have all drawn the same conclusions. Therefore, scientists have mapped-out the expected changes in body composition from bodyweight losses (or gains). This map helps one to understand how to design a diet or exercise program for optimal results.

There are several important questions, here, that we need to ask about bodyweight loss:

1) What is the composition of the weight that's lost during dieting?
2) What are the factors that determine how much fat is lost and how much Lean Body Mass is lost?
3) What is the ratio of Fat Mass loss to Lean Body Mass (muscle and organs) loss?
4) How do different dieting methods affect the expected pattern of loss?

Dr. Gregory Ellis's Ultimate Diet Secrets Lite

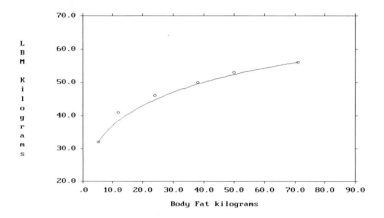

The chart, above, describes the expected relationship between Lean Body Mass loss and Fat Mass loss for a wide range of body fat contents. The vertical line (y-axis) represents the Lean Body Mass (muscles and organs). I'll use the acronym, LBM, for Lean Body Mass from now on.

The horizontal line (x-axis) represents the Fat Mass. The data used to plot the graph represent body types that differ widely in LBM and Fat Mass content. This includes people who are extremely obese to the extremely thin, such as patients with anorexia nervosa.

The shape of the line in the graph is curvilinear. Check it out, see how it curves downward as it moves from right to left. You're actually moving your eyes along the x-axis, from right to left. The x-axis, or horizontal line, is the amount of Fat Mass in kilograms.

This curvilinear shape shows us something important. When a fat person begins a diet, Fat Mass loss is a larger part of the lost bodyweight. In other words, the fat person loses a higher percentage of fat and a smaller percentage of LBM. That's more fat loss and less LBM loss.

In a lean person beginning a diet, less Fat Mass is lost. And he loses more LBM as a part of the total

How Weight Loss (and Gain) Affect Body Composition

bodyweight loss.

You can clearly see this on the curvilinear line. Look at that part of the horizontal line above the 0-30 kilogram points. See how steeply it slopes? Now move your eyes over to the y-axis. This represents the decrease in LBM. See how fast LBM drops here?

Now, look over, on the horizontal line, to the 60-70 Fat Mass kilogram point. You'll see that when one loses fat along this range, there isn't much LBM loss.

The outcome, then, of this curvilinear shape is that the loss of LBM gradually accounts for an ever-increasing proportion of the bodyweight loss as one becomes leaner. This is very interesting and very important to the way weight loss affects you. Later, I'll show you what it all means.

There are dramatic differences, then, for changes in body composition between an obese person and a lean person. The lean person begins the diet with an already smaller amount of Fat Mass. An example would be a boxer, already lean, conditioning for the big fight. As a dieter continues to lose body fat, however, there's a change in the ratio between LBM and Fat Mass losses. This leads to an ever-increasing proportion of the lost bodyweight as LBM. The graph shows, then, that the loss of 10 kilograms of fat by a fat person leads, at the same time, to loss of about 2-3 kilograms of LBM. Conversely, a leaner person losing 7 kilograms of Fat Mass will, at the same time, lose a much higher amount of LBM -- about 7 kilograms. Wow, that's a big difference.

Here's the important information about this fact. Whenever bodyweight loss occurs there's a predictable **"companionship,"** or ratio, between LBM and Fat Mass loss.

This ratio is dependent on the initial Fat Mass of the

dieter registered at the beginning of the diet.

Therefore, the initial amount of Fat Mass determines the early ratio of LBM to Fat Mass loss. In lean individuals, loss of bodyweight results in a larger loss of LBM.

Fat Mass loss becomes less and less of the bodyweight loss the leaner one becomes. So, as Fat Mass decreases, less fat is lost. Yet, at the same time, LBM loss increases.

In the lean, then, bodyweight loss spares fat. Instead, it eats away at the LBM. The body cannibalizes its muscle and organs to provide calories for the muscles, organs, brain, and nervous system. Muscle and organs, then, in a sense, eat themselves the leaner one becomes. For the obese, Fat Mass loss is more of the bodyweight that's lost.

As bodyweight continues to decrease, the body's fat content begins to diminish. At this point, things switch around. The body now tries to protect its fat. It switches over, relying more on the LBM to provide the needed calories.

The body's drive to protect its Fat Mass, however, doesn't become strong until the Fat Mass shrinks a lot, as I'll describe later.

I'll bet that you've never heard any of this before.

Weight Gain

Obese animals or humans can withstand decreased amounts of food, or even starvation, better than lean ones. LBM (Lean Body Mass) and Fat Mass are not independent entities. There's a link between the two, as stated above. Whenever one loses or gains weight, both

How Weight Loss (and Gain) Affect Body Composition

parts of body composition change. And, they change predictably.

Obesity or overweight is always associated with both an increase in Fat Mass and in LBM as well. Fat Mass, though, increases and accounts for the bulk of the weight gain. All parts of the LBM, organs and skeletal muscle, however, increase in size. This is to support and move the increased body mass. Autopsy studies show that obese people have larger hearts, livers, kidneys, spleens, and pancreases than lean people do.

There is a strong relationship between LBM and height. Obesity **distorts** this normal relationship. That's because obese people have more LBM than normal-weight subjects of the same height. The overweight condition, itself, automatically leads to an increase in LBM. This increase in muscles and organs is more than the amount expected for a given height. This is purely a function of becoming overweight.

The LBM increase in obesity accounts for 20-40% of the excess bodyweight increase. The average value for this increase in LBM is about 29%. Scientists believe that the extra LBM causes the increases seen in RMR (Resting Metabolic Rate) in obesity.

Overweight and obese individuals always have an increase in their Total Daily Energy Expenditure (TDEE). Scientists believe that both the increase in bodyweight and in LBM is partly responsible for this.

Humans, who are deliberately overfed, acquire a larger LBM than control subjects who don't overeat. The longest recorded period of controlled overfeeding in human subjects is 83 days.

Does Becoming Overweight or Obese Increase Calorie Needs?

There's a relationship between bodyweight and the calories needed to maintain that weight.

We can plot this relationship in a graph. When we do, we discover the same curvilinear line we saw earlier. The curvilinear line, here, means that weight gain gradually reaches a plateau. Weight gain, at any given calorie amount of overeating eventually slows. Further, as time goes on, weight gain ceases altogether.

This number of calories becomes the new maintenance level for the higher bodyweight!

Calorie needs change as bodyweight increases during overfeeding. For an increase of 2.2 pounds, weight **maintenance** calories increase by about 20 calories a day. This means that a gain of 40 pounds requires eating an additional 400 calories a day to maintain the new weight.

I want to state this again. If the eating of the same excess calories continues, bodyweight increases to a point and then stops. Now, the excess food comes to represent the new **required maintenance** level. If increases in bodyweight continue, through continued overeating, or decreased activity, more of the bodyweight gain is Fat Mass. In contrast, the bodyweight gain that is LBM becomes smaller and smaller as a part of the bodyweight gain.

Here's what happens when leaner, less fat people, overeat. Their bodyweight gain, in the early stages, is more LBM and less Fat Mass. For example, anorexia nervosa patients' increases in LBM represent 68% of their **early** bodyweight gains.

Therefore, people recovering from famine, or those

ending a diet, have rapid increases in LBM in the early stages of eating more food. Fat Mass increases represent less of the bodyweight gain during the early stages of more normal eating.

These proportions change, however, as formerly food-restricted individuals approach their previous, normal bodyweight. During this phase, the proportion of the tissue increase that is Fat Mass **outpaces** the early, more rapid, increases in LBM. The accumulating Fat Mass gain, then, continues to climb, faster and higher, than the gain in LBM.

Experiments show that the increases in Fat Mass continue because the person fails to slow down food intake. Hunger turns-on, a natural, well known consequence of long-term reduced-food intake.

What's the result? The Fat Mass **overshoots** its original, normal level. We term this effect "**post-starvation obesity**."

This is the precise reason why many people gain more bodyweight than they lost upon ending a diet. The body is aggressive in trying to restore its lost weight. This includes both the LBM and Fat Mass. The body turns-on powerful physiological drives that push hunger and appetite. It revs them into high gear whose purpose is to re-build the lost tissues.

This is why you must have a thorough understanding of all of the mechanisms involved in the total weight control picture. This is the only way you can use effective **counter-strategies**, the only way to avoid the inevitable "**post-diet obesity**" occurring with weight loss programs.

Weight Loss

Weight loss leads to changes in both the Fat Mass

and the LBM. And again, the primary factor determining the ratio between the two is the amount of the pre-diet Fat Mass.

I'm going to give you a confusing sentence, but then I'll explain what it means. Here it is. The ratio between LBM and change in bodyweight is 0.27 for an obese individual and 0.46 for a lean, non-obese one. Here's the explanation. For one who is obese this ratio means that for every pound of bodyweight that's lost, 27% of that one pound loss is LBM. And 73% of the loss is Fat Mass. For one who is lean, the loss of one pound is represented by a 46% LBM loss and a 54% loss in Fat Mass.

It's helpful to understand that these ratios vary. This depends on the Fat Mass registered at the beginning of the diet. So, when starting a weight loss program, expect an ever-changing ratio of LBM to Fat Mass loss as bodyweight decreases.

You must understand these predictable changes. This way you can have a strategic plan in place to prevent losses in LBM, particularly in the muscle component of the LBM. An understanding of these relationships also helps one avoid the post-dieting gains in Fat Mass.

I'll teach you such a strategy. It's one that's guaranteed to modify the normally-expected changes. With this technique in hand, you can minimize LBM losses and maximize Fat Mass losses!

Lean Body Mass Changes

Current research shows that there's no level of reduced energy intake that completely spares LBM when losing weight.

This isn't always true, though, if you know what you're doing. I do, and I'll prove it to you later on when I

How Weight Loss (and Gain) Affect Body Composition

tell you about my own research and experiments.

Even modest reductions in calorie intake lead to some loss of LBM. In one study, adult men reduced their intake of calories by 500 each day below the usual amount. Over a period of 70 days, they lost 6 kilograms. About 33% of the loss consisted of LBM.

In the previous chapter, I described my experiences with the VLCD (Very Low Calorie Diet). I described the efforts of scientists to construct a "protein-sparing" (LBM preserving) diet.

Needless to say, people and medical doctors were enamored with the VLCD because of the rapid weight loss experienced by users. Its downside, however, was the rapid decrease in Resting Metabolic Rate (RMR). This was because of the rapid decreases in LBM. And, as we'll see later, the VLCD drives changes in the cells "metabolic efficiency." These changes occurred particularly in the big calorie users such as the liver. Consequently, the researchers determined that the calories of the VLCD should comprise high-quality proteins.

They believed that these high-quality proteins would spare the LBM, reducing its rate of loss. This modification was, however, only partly successful. This was because the calorie deficiency, itself, overwhelmed any positive effect of the high-protein VLCD.

Fasting, the complete absence of food, leads, obviously, to the most rapid losses in both LBM and Fat Mass. Food, even small amounts, such as 400 calories a day, slows this loss. It does not, though, completely spare LBM loss.

Maintenance of LBM is dependent upon an adequate calorie intake. Therefore, the amount of LBM loss depends upon the amount of the calorie reduction. And, again, as we'll see, on diet composition too.

It's important for you to construct a bodyweight loss plan that's based on these facts to optimize bodyweight loss and LBM preservation.

The graph, below, clearly demonstrates the effect of differing levels of calorie intake on the ratio of LBM to Fat Mass loss. The -- line represents the expected ratio of LBM to Fat Mass loss. This line, of course, is dependent upon initial Fat Mass.

The star symbol represents a range of calorie intake between 0-440 per day (typical of a VLCD). This extreme method of calorie reduction leads to an average loss of about 50% LBM.

The light circles represent a calorie intake of 500-900 a day. A diet containing this number of calories leads to less LBM loss (about 30% of the bodyweight loss) and more Fat Mass loss. See how this compares to a calorie intake of less than 500 per day?

How Weight Loss (and Gain) Affect Body Composition

Diets of 1,000-1,400 calories a day are marked by the square symbols. These show that the ratio of the loss of the two tissues follows the expected line. The dark-edged circles represent 1,500-1,900 calories per day. These points indicate that a slower rate of loss leads to a preservation of LBM while increasing the loss of Fat Mass.

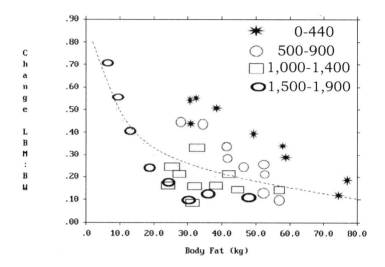

The trend for all the diets, varying in daily calorie content, follows this expected line.

But, there are potential disruptors to this trend. They arise from 1) the rate of weight loss and 2) the calorie content of the diet. These factors, obviously, are dependent on each other. They also depend, as you know by now, of course, on the initial amount of Fat Mass.

The implication of this chart for you is that as the total Fat Mass decreases, further bodyweight losses involve a higher proportion of LBM. Fat mass loss slows and LBM loss increases.

We can, however, use techniques to modify these predictable changes.

In summary, why is this information important to you? There's a take-home message from these sections, above. It's that, **whenever** one loses bodyweight, both LBM and Fat Mass are parts (varying) of the loss.

These two body parts, therefore, are **companions**. A change in one is accompanied by a change in the other. They are not independent entities. The initial Fat Mass of an individual when beginning to lose weight is a critical factor in determining the **composition** of the initial tissue loss. It also determines the **ratio** of tissue loss too.

Understanding these facts is important to finding and using methods that trip-up these predictable changes. The use of these methods will benefit you. These methods, that I'll describe, force the body away from the expected ratio of LBM to Fat Mass loss.

They drive it to **maximize** losses in fat, while **minimizing** losses in LBM.

These methods can even force the body to increase LBM while losing fat!

This is particularly important as one becomes leaner. This is because, as we've learned, a decreasing Fat Mass **automatically** causes the body to lose a higher proportion of LBM.

These are **Very Powerful Techniques** if they can modify and alter the body's automatic regulatory systems.

This is the first time in the history of the weight loss and weight control business that such a comprehensive program is now available. It took me over 40 years to understand, develop, and refine my program.

There's nothing that's even remotely close to my system.

Water Losses

It's important now to discuss weight loss relative to the percentage of lost bodyweight that's water. This is extremely important to the dieter who has been besieged by a glut of weight loss programs. These programs were designed by unscrupulous marketers who "promise" stupendous bodyweight losses to those purchasing their programs.

All the explanations, above, concerning the ratio of the loss of the two different body parts, LBM and Fat Mass, are changes occurring over a long time. So any influence from other variables, such as water, is minimal. In the early days of a weight loss program, however, the story is entirely different.

Below are two tables that show the results of two different experiments in human semi-starvation studies. They demonstrate the consistent finding of an early and rapid loss of bodyweight composed mostly of water and not Fat Mass.

Days of Semi-Starvation	1-3	4-6	7-12
Avg. Weight Loss/Day			
Kilograms	0.73	0.50	0.37
Pounds	1.61	1.10	0.81
Fat % loss	27	40	53
LBM % loss	9	10	13
Water % loss	64	50	34

Days of Semi-Starvation	1-3	11-13	22-24
Avg. Weight Loss/Day			
Kilograms	0.80	0.23	0.31
Pounds	1.76	0.50	0.14
Fat % loss	25	69	85
LBM % loss	5	12	15
Water % loss	70	19	0

These two charts provide an excellent description of the changes in water weight in the body's response to semi-starvation. In these studies, there was a reduction by 50% in daily calorie intake.

During the 1st-3rd days, bodyweight loss is dramatic. This is similar to the weight loss experienced by most people when beginning a diet. All of these people believe, of course, that their weight loss was fat tissue. What a mistake!

As you can see, in studying the tables, the percentage of bodyweight lost in the first three days is 70% water. Fat Mass loss represents only 25-27% of the total bodyweight loss!

As the semi-starvation period continues, the **rate** of bodyweight loss rapidly decreases. This is because the losses of water are decreasing. They continue to decrease until 22-24 days. By this time, water loss ceases completely.

This is consistent with the time, in most dietary protocols, when massive frustration sets in for the unsuspecting dieter. This is because their weight loss has slowed to a trickle. It's then that he realizes that he's been taken to the cleaners. He's been lied to by the weight loss scam artists who flood the marketplace and the media.

How Weight Loss (and Gain) Affect Body Composition

Lose 30 pounds in 30 days! Call me Now!

And what's most shocking is that the gullible public buys into this, over and over and over.

Changes in Body Composition

It's important to remember that the calculations presented in earlier pages, arising from data in the accompanying graphs, are dependent upon several factors, as we've seen. These include the amount of calorie restriction, the physical activity level, and the initial Fat Mass registered before beginning a diet. These calculations, though, vary depending upon where you are on the LBM/Fat Mass ratio line. They also vary to the degree of changes in any factor or combination of these factors, above.

Much of the information, above, was first presented in scientific publications in the late 1980's. When I was undergoing my body composition experiments while on the complex carbohydrate diet, I wasn't aware of these established relationships.

Unbeknownst to me, I was actually participating in and adding to the scientific base by my own confirmatory experiments. Every increase in my bodyweight followed the line plotted in the graph, above. There was a 25% increase in bodyweight represented by LBM and a 75% increase in bodyweight represented by Fat Mass.

Conversely, my attempts at slimming always resulted in exactly the same ratio of changes. I experienced a loss of 75% in Fat Mass and a loss of 25% in LBM. I wasn't at the extreme ends of the line: I was neither too fat nor too lean. And, for that reason, my changes followed the predictions dictated by the midpoint of the line, depicted on the graph. If I'd been at one extreme or the other, the ratio would have been different, as the graph predicts.

My bodyweight changes, up and down were always accompanied by changes in my body composition. These followed the line as shown in the graph.

I wanted, obviously, to gain more muscle and lose more fat as a result of my diet changes. The complex carbohydrate diet, however, failed to effect any alteration in the expected ratio: my body followed the line as shown on the graph.

This diet composition, therefore, was not the grand strategic method. It wasn't the dietary regimen I'd been led to believe would provide more muscle while, at the same time, reduce fat.

These facts fueled my future explorations. I wanted desperately to identify exercise or dietary modifications that could alter this all-important ratio in the direction I desired. I wanted more muscle tissue and less Fat Mass on my body. Scientists, of course, have learned that using anabolic steroids is effective in altering the ratio. However, I had a negative experience with steroids and, as a consequence, they weren't an option.

My experiments confirmed the failure of the complex carbohydrate diet. They also confirmed that the weight lifting methods I'd recently used were not a stimulus for further muscle growth either. Certainly, I knew that increasing my calorie intake (and bodyweight) would increase my LBM. Yet, the simultaneously occurring downside was that this would also increase my Fat Mass. I needed to make further **refinements** in both my diet and exercise program to elicit the changes that I desired.

Another question I had, however, was whether I'd already reached my genetic limits and, hence, reached a point of no further improvements.

I wasn't yet ready to resign myself to that possibility.

How Weight Loss (and Gain) Affect Body Composition

The graphs, above, plot the average, expected changes occurring in an individual in the process of either losing or gaining bodyweight.

Energy Partitioning

Energy-partitioning says that fuel is diverted into the active tissues and burned for energy, or, it's diverted into the adipose tissue where it remains as a reserve source of energy. This is not an all or none proposition; these processes occur at the same time.

But if the rate of energy-partitioning into fat tissue exceeds the amount that is burned in the active tissues, then overweight and increases in Fat Mass become the inevitable result.

Enzymes control energy-partitioning. Enzymes can increase or decrease, in both **quantity** and **activity**, through signals provided by the nervous and endocrine systems. The stimuli to these responses arise from changes in food quantity, food composition, and physical activity.

My early research into uncovering these facts, combined with my more detailed research into fuel metabolism for my Ph. D. dissertation, led me, as I've stated, into my next major area of exploration: the low-carbohydrate diet, a diet that we'll explore shortly.

Dr. Gregory Ellis's Ultimate Diet Secrets Lite

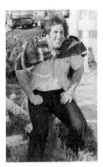
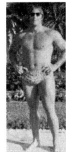
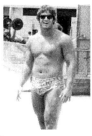
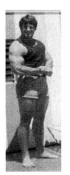
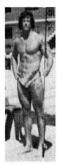

250 pounds

245 pounds California 1970

235 pounds right before San Diego Chargers camp, 1970

222 pounds Fall 1970

216 pounds summer 1972

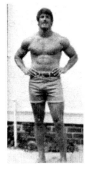
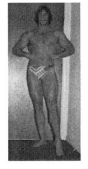
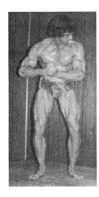
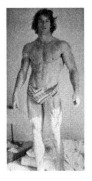

207 pounds summer 1969

205 pounds Fall 1972

192 pounds summer 1973

After 1st Pep-up, 185 pounds

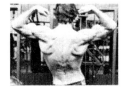

175 pounds winter 1975

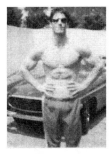

~ 175 lbs

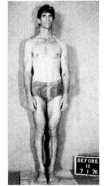

165 pounds post-fasting 1976

How Weight Loss (and Gain) Affect Body Composition

By the late 1970's, I'd completed extensive experiments in changing my body. I'd experienced the most extreme gains and losses in weight imaginable. By 1976, when I fasted, I lost all my fat, and because I continued to starve myself, I lost all my hard-earned muscles too. As you look at the photos you can see how muscle and fat are companions in the weight loss process.

Metabolic Adaptations

But, before going into the low-carbohydrate diet, I want to follow-up on the exposition, above, about body composition. I want to provide you with a detailed analysis of what has been one of the most exciting discoveries of my more than 43 years of studying weight control. I'm going to devote some time to discuss the subject of "Metabolic Adaptations" here. My full understanding of the mechanisms underlying Metabolic Adaptations has occurred only recently, during the last two years.

My early experiences with Metabolic Adaptations were adaptations that prevented further bodyweight losses or gains during my dietary experiments. They forced me to eat sparingly to maintain the lower bodyweight and low fat percent I'd achieved. Those same adaptations prevented further bodyweight gain even with the consumption of enormous amounts of food when I reached 265 pounds.

I knew that something was going on, but didn't understand it. Now I do.

Here's the most important reason, however, to discuss this topic thoroughly, here, rather than later. It's that a full understanding of Metabolic Adaptations is necessary to an understanding of the discussions yet to come about diet composition, exercise, and the integrated weight loss and weight control program that I've developed.

My programs are effective for anyone wanting to lose weight. This is true for a 300-pounder trying to lose weight, or for an athlete or bodybuilder trying to optimize his or her body for sports performance. The underlying principles are similar. There are, however, important changes that occur depending upon a multitude of varying factors that I'll lay out for you.

A lean body operates according to far different dynamics than a fat body. One must know the level at which he or she is operating in order to fulfill completely his goals. This becomes increasingly more difficult, however, because the leaner one becomes, the more the rules change. You'll need to know exactly how to change your weight loss program in order to achieve success when confronted with these rule changes. That's because weight loss changes the way the body burns calories. Let's now see how the body adapts to changes in food intake and weight change.

How the Body's Metabolism Adapts to Dieting and Weight Loss

I've wrestled long and hard trying to decide how to rank the importance of the information in this section. I didn't come to a thorough understanding of Metabolic Adaptations until the year 2000. In short, Metabolic Adaptations are changes that occur in the body in response to food availability and bodyweight changes. Metabolic Adaptations change metabolism, the way the body uses calories. The amount of changes in body composition determines the extent of Metabolic Adaptations.

My experiences led me to think that Metabolic Adaptations might be the most important factor in solving problems in weight loss and weight control. I found it difficult, though, to accept that idea. I'd placed so much emphasis on the **primary** importance of the

How Weight Loss (and Gain) Affect Body Composition

Energy Balance Equation that I figured nothing would control it.

I thought about my dilemma for several months. Then, it finally struck me that these two seemingly **independent** issues -- the Energy Balance Equation and Metabolic Adaptations -- were, in fact, unified. They were not, in any sense, **independent** of one another. Metabolic Adaptations are, simply, adaptations that happen within and as a part of the Energy Balance Equation.

As I've told you, I directly experienced the effects of Metabolic Adaptations during my overfeeding and underfeeding studies. When I was younger I reached a personal high bodyweight of 265 pounds. Here, I found it impossible to consume enough food to maintain that ponderous body mass. In another experiment to decrease bodyweight, I reached 165 pounds. Here, I found it just as impossible to maintain that personal low bodyweight.

At a bodyweight of 165 pounds, I ate sparingly. This was sharply in contrast with the 10,000 calories a day that I'd consumed at 265 pounds. Throughout the following decades, I always found it rather easy to maintain a bodyweight of 220 pounds. I "settled" easily into this weight while consuming an amount of food that was satisfying. I was fatter at 220 pounds, though, than I wanted to be. So, I would reduce my food intake to lose some fat. Every time I tried to push my weight to a lower level, I required an ever-lower level of calories to reach my goal. That fact was indisputable.

This observation made me question the simplistic calculations used by nutritionists in weight loss programs. They first measure the subject's bodyweight, then they calculate his calorie needs based on standardized tables. They use the Body Mass Index (BMI) or measure the subject's body composition to figure out his ideal bodyweight and then calculate the number of calories the subject needs to eat to reduce to a new lower bodyweight. They use the assumption that each pound of fat contains 3,500 calories.

They make **no provision** for the fact that a portion of the lost bodyweight will include a loss of Lean Body Mass (muscles and organs, see the previous section on body composition).

And, they make **no provision**, in short, for the Metabolic Adaptations I'm about to describe.

This time-worn procedure is overly simplistic. It's doomed to fail because the nutritionist makes **no provision** for the fact that, as one sheds pounds, Metabolic Adaptations occur. These Adaptations lead to fewer pounds lost at the same calorie intake. In other words, one loses weight (and fat) faster the fatter one is. As one becomes "leaner," this process changes dramatically. For example, let's say we reduce one's calorie intake by 1,000 calories a day. Over time, this reduced calorie intake will fail to stimulate the same rate of bodyweight loss as it did at the start of the diet.

Again, a decrease in calorie intake below energy needs results in more weight loss the fatter one is. It also leads to more fat loss. As the diet proceeds and bodyweight decreases, the **rate** of bodyweight loss will slow or even stop. **It's very important that this fundamental fact is understood!**

It's assumed that each pound of fat is worth 3,500 calories, as I've said. Under this assumption, a decrease in daily calorie intake of 500 would, theoretically, lead to a loss of one pound per week. That's because 7 days times 500 calories a day equals 3,500 calories, the assumed energy content of one pound of fat. One could also accomplish the same effect by burning 500 more

How Weight Loss (and Gain) Affect Body Composition

calories a day.

By following such a program for 12 weeks, the calculation **predicts** that the bodyweight loss will be 12 pounds. This is how the weight loss "experts" calculate potential losses. Further, everyone assumes that the bodyweight loss is composed solely of fat. This is a monumentally mistaken assumption!

What are the two mistaken assumptions? First, that reducing calories leads to a continuous, steady loss of bodyweight for a given amount of calorie reduction. And second, that the lost bodyweight is composed entirely of fat tissue. Both assumptions are wrong.

This section is all about the failure of these assumptions. These assumptions must be modified. The new assumptions must embrace the changes that occur in the body because of weight loss and food restriction. I term these changes Metabolic Adaptations (not to be confused with the erroneous Atkins phrase "metabolic advantage").

My discussion, therefore, is to present the facts about how the body changes when stressed by food deprivation. I'll tell you about the changes from varying calorie intakes and I'll also tell you about how changes in bodyweight, Fat Mass, and Lean Body Mass affect Metabolic Adaptations.

My own weight loss experiences didn't follow the expected calorie-cutting, straight-line weight loss theory. Further, my bodyweight loss was never composed exclusively of fat, but of both Fat Mass and Lean Body Mass.

Therefore, the belief that a simple calorie reduction causes a loss of bodyweight composed solely of fat is false. I remember that for years I questioned these beliefs. My own experiences were inconsistent with these assumptions. I told this to friends and training buddies. There was something seriously amiss with the "Just reduce your calories and you'll reach your target weight" theory.

It was clear to me that losing bodyweight became more and more difficult the **leaner** I became. I had always experienced that. For me, it was much easier to go from 220 to 210 pounds than from 195 to 190. Because of Metabolic Adaptations, it's easy for a 250 pound, 40% fat individual to reduce his bodyweight to, say, 210 pounds at 30% fat. For someone leaner, it's much more difficult to reduce. As a result, an already lean 200 pound, 10% fat individual has a hard time reducing his bodyweight to 190 pounds at 8% fat.

All of this implies that there is some type of increase in **"metabolic efficiency"** occurring during bodyweight reduction. This metabolic efficiency allows an individual to **"extract"** more energy from each calorie consumed. Yet, in spite of my experiences, I'd never heard any discussion of these ideas. I thought I was nuts because I had always been taught that "a calorie is a calorie is a calorie."

Earlier, I explained this idea. A calorie is a calorie and has, by definition, a precise amount of energy, a scientific fact, beyond dispute. So what then is going on? The only conclusion that one can reach is that adaptations must occur **within** the body itself. The body must then perform all its functions while consuming less energy. This, then, effectively makes each calorie go further. Wow!

And, this is precisely what happens: the body now functions adequately by using less fuel! Unearthing this fact solved the problem of bodyweight changes not accommodating themselves to the accepted model. It gives rise, of course, to many new and interesting questions about how the body adapts. One unanswered question is whether the new functional level is just as healthy as the previous functional level? Science doesn't yet have answers to these questions because the study of Metabolic Adaptations has barely scratched the surface. (There are, however, a significant number of animal studies showing that food restriction increases life-span and health. Intriguing.)

But, let's talk about what <u>we do know</u> and how that information is of paramount importance in the success of your weight loss and weight control program.

First, however, I have to review several terms that we've discussed in previous chapters. **This is because these body processes are the ones affected by Metabolic Adaptations.**

Resting Metabolic Rate (RMR) is the amount of calories required by the body to maintain its daily obligated functions. This is the "stay-alive" energy required by the body. The Thermic Effect of Food (TEF) is the amount of calories used by the body to digest food. Although Metabolic Adaptations do affect TEF, these changes aren't significant. Therefore, in the intent of economy, we won't consider the impact of Metabolic Adaptations on TEF.

Physical Activity Level (PAL) is the number of calories used to move the body around each day. Total Daily Energy Expenditure (TDEE) is the total amount of calories burned by an individual for a 24-hour period.

TDEE is the sum of the Resting Metabolic Rate (RMR) and the Physical Activity Level (PAL). For an average individual, RMR represents about 65-70% of the TDEE (total calories burned each day). PAL represents about

20-25% of TDEE. The Thermic Effect of Food represents about 10% of the TDEE.

Obviously, the most variable factor is PAL, with some people's Physical Activity Level (PAL) matching, or even exceeding, their RMR. Here's an example. If a person's RMR is 1,750 calories a day, a very active person may expend another 1,750 calories in his daily physical activity. It's well-established that most persons' TDEEs are approximately 1.5-1.6 times their Resting Metabolic Rate (RMR). A very active person's Total Daily Energy Expenditure (TDEE) may be 2-2.5 times his Resting Metabolic Rate (RMR).

So, the **two primary parts** of one's energy expenditure are RMR and PAL. Their sum is TDEE (I'm skipping the Thermic Effect of Food, about 10% of the TDEE). Metabolic Adaptations affect RMR and PAL and, hence, affect TDEE, the sum of RMR and PAL.

Changes in body composition affect Metabolic Adaptations. One of the important players, here, is the Lean Body Mass (LBM). LBM is the muscles and organs. The other player is the Fat Mass (adipose tissue). Fat Mass represents the stored energy reserves of the body.

Food restriction, **decreased or increased bodyweight**, and **changes in body composition** are the "environmental stresses" leading to Metabolic Adaptations. Metabolic Adaptations, in turn, affect the main players: RMR, PAL, TDEE, Fat Mass, and Lean Body Mass. The body's response to these "environmental stresses" is determined by changes in control messages arising from the nervous system and the hormonal system. They, in turn, tell the tissues of the body how to respond.

How Weight Loss (and Gain) Affect Body Composition

What are the Effects of Overfeeding

A very large proportion of the population believes that some people can eat a lot of food without gaining weight. They believe that other people, just sniffing food, gain weight easily. This belief is held by "experts" and lay people alike. In short, they believe that people can maintain a constant bodyweight while eating a diet that varies widely in calories. Let's review this more closely.

As in the underfeeding studies, above, overfeeding leads to similar responses. The **observed** bodyweight increase during overfeeding is always less than **predicted**. Therefore, underfeeding results in less bodyweight **loss** than expected and, on the other hand, overfeeding results in less bodyweight **gain** than expected.

The body converts food not used for immediate energy into body fat. The production of and maintenance of the body tissues requires the expenditure of energy. The body must use calories to make new tissues and to maintain them.

Therefore, the body uses calories to store excess food as body fat. The maintenance of muscles and organs also requires the use of calories and this conversion of food into fat raises heat production and metabolic rate.

In a previous section I've shown that as Fat Mass increases, Lean Body Mass also increases. Further, a higher bodyweight demands the use of more calories just to move around the increased weight. Storage of food as fat, the building of muscles and organs, and the increased bodyweight consume calories. As Fat Mass, Lean Body Mass, (and, of course, bodyweight) increase, calorie expenditure increases. Together, this calorie demand consumes some of the extra food from overfeeding, reducing the number of calories available to increase bodyweight.

This fact is in conflict with the idea of **luxuskonsumption** that the body takes **all** of the extra calories it consumes during overfeeding and converts them to heat, avoiding any weight gain.

There's a major limitation to research in this area. It's that changes in bodyweight aren't good indicators of energy gains or losses over short periods.

Studies of overfeeding (or underfeeding) must be extended for as long as possible. The reason is to reduce errors stemming from the variable changes in bodyweight. These changes may come from variations in, say, body water content. Further, there are individual variations from overfeeding or underfeeding and these individual responses make analysis from these types of studies difficult. For example, there are subjects who store body fat a little more easily than others.

In summary, adaptations to variations in calorie intake prevent the **predicted** bodyweight changes during low calorie or high calorie eating. As a result, bodyweight changes are **always** less than **predicted**.

Also, when bodyweight increases, there's always an increase in calorie intake. The higher bodyweight requires additional calories to support it and this becomes the new maintenance intake for the higher bodyweight. In contrast, the calorie needs to support a lower bodyweight are always **fewer** than they were to support the before-weight loss bodyweight.

An individual's Total Daily Energy Expenditure (TDEE) always decreases during a period of a too low calorie intake. TDEE is always lower after a drop in bodyweight. TDEE can only remain at the higher level previous to weight loss if the individual increases it by consciously adding physical activity (PAL). Conversely, the opposite happens with a high calorie intake. Under this condition of increased bodyweight, TDEE increases. Daily calorie intake also increases to meet energy needs. These include both the increased bodyweight and calorie cost of making fat and muscle. Most of the additional calorie use arises as a result of the calories needed to carry around the increased bodyweight.

Set-Point Theory of Bodyweight

Every person appears to have a Set-Point for bodyweight. This is a set bodyweight toward which the body naturally gravitates. We've learned that bodyweight is highly regulated by in-born balancing controls, controls that act automatically and are highly regulated. They help the body to respond to forces pushing it away from its Set-Point. These controls are part of the body's effort to maintain life in the face of challenges to its survival.

Body composition, particularly Fat Mass, is a primary factor in the control of Metabolic Adaptations. Increases or decreases in Fat Mass stimulate fat tissue to release a signal, as yet unknown, that affects appetite and hunger. The signal also affects physical activity patterns. Through changes in hormones and nervous system activity, both Resting Metabolic Rate (RMR) and Physical Activity Level (PAL) automatically change. These two, RMR and PAL, are the two parts of the Total Daily Energy Expenditure (TDEE).

Hormonal changes and input from the nervous system drive the body's adaptations. They influence enzymes that control fuel use. Fuel is either burned for energy or stored in the fat tissue as an energy reserve. Fat Mass appears to have the strongest control over the strength of the Metabolic Adaptations in comparison to Lean Body Mass. Studies into these mechanisms, however, are still in their infancy.

Metabolic and behavioral forces resist changes in both bodyweight and body composition. As an individual moves away from his in-born Set-Point, powerful forces push him to return to it. These automatic bodyweight controls include ***involuntary*** changes in food intake and physical activity patterns. Further, shifts in heat production caused by changes in hormones and the sympathetic nervous system work together to maintain pre-existing bodyweight.

Many reduced formerly-obese individuals, in spite of maintaining their weight loss, suffer a myriad of symptoms. These include a sense of unrest, depression, cold intolerance, hunger, and menstrual dysfunction. Interestingly, these are the same symptoms associated with fasting. These responses are compatible, in short, with individuals suffering from starvation.

Studies into all the factors involved in these observations are few. Clearly, the observed symptom complex, including the reduction in calorie needs, serves as a potent force pushing the body to regain the lost Fat Mass.

I argue, however, that both physical activity and diet composition control several of the powerful metabolic factors involved in pushing weight regain. Later, in my discussion of these two factors, I'll show that performing a "threshold" amount of physical activity and eating the right type of foods minimize the power of these forces.

The strength of these forces is directly proportional to how far the body moves away from its Set-Point. This includes its Set-Point for bodyweight and particularly for body composition. These forces, attempting to restore the body to its original Set-Point, behave like a coiled spring. The spring's tension increases as the distance from the resting point increases. The forces tending to return the spring to its coiled Set-Point become stronger the more it's uncoiled. Similarly, the forces to return bodyweight to its Set-Point become stronger the more bodyweight moves, in either direction, from its Set-Point.

We don't need to understand all the mechanisms before we use these controls for our benefit. The failure to understand this truism has caused countless weight loss and weight control failures.

Nonetheless, it's now well-established that the Energy Balance Equation is valid. Each side of the equation, Calories-In (the food one eats) and Calories-Out (the calories one burns), is affected powerfully by changes in food intake and physical activity. Changes in both the absolute and relative amounts of the two body tissues: Lean Body Mass (muscles and organs) and Fat Mass also affect food intake and physical activity.

How Do Changes in Food Intake Affect the Two Main Parts of Calorie Burn?

The human body responds to a lowered food intake by a large number of complex responses. These responses represent stress adaptations to a reduced calorie intake and are, as a consequence, survival mechanisms.

A decrease in bodyweight is a constant, and most obvious outcome, of a reduced calorie intake. A reduction in calories can be self-imposed for purposes of weight loss or it's an involuntary consequence of famine or some such dislocation of nature.

In the previous section, I discussed extensively the changes in the two main parts of body composition, Lean Body Mass and Fat Mass, in response to calorie restriction.

We must understand the **calorie-sparing adaptations** resulting from reduced food intake that are consequent to the loss of bodyweight. This understanding is important to a successful and effective weight loss and weight control program. Fundamentally, the weight loss portion is usually the easiest part of the weight loss and weight control effort. People simply reduce their food intake for a time, and they lose weight.

The most difficult part of the process, however, is the maintenance of the new bodyweight.

This process is made all the more difficult because there's rarely ever a discussion about the influence of Metabolic Adaptations. In my own case, I didn't understand the impact of Metabolic Adaptations until I'd invested more than 40 years of effort into weight control.

No one and no program ever discussed the importance of this issue. Most commercial programs always emphasize the **ease** of following their program, guaranteeing success **without any effort** on the part of the dieter. A present-day diet guru tells us that, by following her program, you'll just melt the fat away. That statement is so contrary to the actual facts that it's impossible to believe other statements about the "dietary science" presented by this author (Suzanne Somers).

The first, and immediate, response of the body to a decrease in food intake is a decrease in calorie burn. This occurs to both Resting Metabolic Rate (RMR) and the Physical Activity Level (PAL); the sum of these two parts is, as we've learned, the Total Daily Energy Expenditure (TDEE).

The important question is, What is the individual contribution of changes in RMR and in Physical Activity Level (PAL) to the overall changes in the body's calorie-sparing adaptations?

How Weight Loss (and Gain) Affect Body Composition

A common finding with reduced food intake is an immediate decrease in RMR. Studies have shown that RMR decreases by almost 5% on the very first day of beginning a diet. This drop can even be more than 5%, depending on the amount of reduction in calorie intake. Continuation of the diet leads to further decreases in RMR. The amount of the RMR drop depends on several factors. These include the level of calorie restriction, the length of the diet, the amount of bodyweight loss, and the changes in body composition.

The decrease in Resting Metabolic Rate (RMR) occurs in several distinct Phases. The initial Phase, Phase 1, occurs during the first 2-3 weeks of food restriction. Here, there is a marked decrease in RMR not accounted for solely by the loss of bodyweight.

We use the term "active tissue" to designate the tissues of the body that consume the most calories. It's well-established that the Lean Body Mass is the highest consumer of calories. But, Lean Body Mass contains both muscles and organs. And of these two, it's the organs, particularly the liver and central nervous system, that consume the most calories.

Skeletal muscles are low calorie consumers until they are used. So resting skeletal muscle consumes few calories. Therefore, the Phase 1 decrease in RMR is represented by a decrease in the RMR of the active tissue mass. This is particularly true for the organs. It's important to understand that this decrease in RMR isn't because of a decrease in tissue weight. These tissues now, simply, need fewer calories to maintain their function as an adaptive response to calorie restriction.

This decrease is an "active process" and we consider it a measure of the increase in "metabolic efficiency" of the active tissue mass. This represents the primary form of Metabolic Adaptation. **The decrease in the cellular** *calorie use begins to level off. It, nonetheless, continues as long as one continues to lose bodyweight, particularly Fat Mass.*

We've learned that the primary determinant of RMR is the Lean Body Mass (muscles and organs, but especially organs). We've now learned that there's a change in the calorie need of the tissues independent of any change in their weight.

In the Minnesota Study, 66% of the decrease in RMR was **independent** of the change in the weight of the Lean Body Mass. Scientists accept that there is a very tight relationship between Lean Body Mass and RMR.

Why, then, did this expected tight relationship fall apart under the conditions imposed on the participants of the Minnesota Study?

It fell apart because of Metabolic Adaptations demonstrating the powerful changes occurring within the **cells** as they adapt to decreased food availability.

This process is wholly demonstrated in a comparison of anorexia nervosa patients with normal individuals of similar Lean Body Mass. Anorexia patients suffer a decrease in RMR that isn't explained by the decrease in Lean Body Mass. This demonstrates an increased metabolic efficiency within the cells, a response to a significant reduction in food intake. Such observations force us to account for these adaptations when the body deviates significantly from its Set-Point.

The adaptation in Phase 2 occurs because of the actual decrease in the bodyweight. Now, it takes fewer calories to move this smaller bodyweight around. This **decrease** in calorie needs continues to grow as long as one continues to lose bodyweight. Therefore, the overall decrease in calorie needs during Phase 2 is **dependent** upon the amount of bodyweight loss.

How Weight Loss (and Gain) Affect Body Composition

This is a different factor than a change in metabolic efficiency. Phase 2 is a "passive process," in contrast to Phase 1's "active process." During Phase 2, the body consumes its own tissues to meet the energy deficit from calorie intake reduction.

The decreased energy need as a consequence of decreases in bodyweight is obvious. One simply has less weight to carry around and, hence, less work to do. Less bodyweight means less work, requiring the consumption of fewer calories.

The decreased calorie need arising from increased metabolic efficiency is <u>not obvious. Thus, there's rarely a discussion about it</u>. Nonetheless, it's a consequence, always, of decreased food intake and losses in bodyweight. No matter the method that one chooses -- whether low-fat or low-carbohydrate, whatever -- the loss of bodyweight always results in Metabolic Adaptations in which the body spares calorie use.

Decreases in calorie burn during Phase 1 include adaptations aimed at reducing the cell's calorie needs. These adaptations are wide-ranging. They affect the body at its very deepest levels. The study of these mechanisms is relatively new, at this juncture. We know very little about the actual changes involved.

But we do know, at the whole body level, how these changes affect our requirements for calories.

Many of the studies into Metabolic Adaptations have been performed on obese subjects. This is because of the necessity to help solve the obesity epidemic. Scientists have performed far fewer studies on normal weight individuals undergoing food restriction. Normal weight individuals, however, demonstrate Metabolic Adaptations similar to the changes experienced by obese subjects undergoing a weight loss program. In fact, the strength of these changes in normal weight individuals is usually greater.

Here's the important point. The obese and normal weight individual start losing weight at different places on their Set-Point and LBM/Fat Mass continuums in respect to both bodyweight and body composition.

The obese individual has moved upward beyond his Set-Point. The body's forces constantly try to push bodyweight back, downward to the original Set-Point. In contrast, the normal weight individual, undergoing a weight loss regimen, moves downward, away from his Set-Point. The body's forces resist this downward deflection. They vigorously try to push bodyweight upward.

These facts show that it's much easier for an overweight individual to reduce downward to his Set-Point because the body wants to drop down to its Set-Point anyway. Conversely, it's much more difficult for a normal weight individual to reduce below his Set-Point. The forces acting to restore his weight become much stronger as the bodyweight decreases in an already lean person and these forces are related to the loss of Lean Body Mass (muscles and organs) and also of Fat Mass.

In the Minnesota Study, normal weight volunteers were reduced in bodyweight by 25%. Recent research about this study shows that the decreasing Fat Mass is the most powerful stimulator of Metabolic Adaptations. Decreases in Fat Mass are the strongest driver of the forces that attempt to drive weight regain. Therefore, the leaner one becomes, the more difficult it is to become yet leaner. The amount of calorie-sparing is powerfully determined by the amount of the tissue loss (both Fat Mass and Lean Body Mass). It's important to understand

How Weight Loss (and Gain) Affect Body Composition

that **reduced food intake** and **tissue loss** work together in determining the strength of Metabolic Adaptations.

The term that represents the measurable decreases (or increases) in calorie needs is thermogenesis. This is a measure of the heat production of the body.

The strong signals arising from the loss of the Fat Mass represent, to me, a third Phase of Metabolic Adaptations. This 3rd Phase relates **strictly** to the amount of the loss in the Fat Mass and Lean Body Mass. This fact has very important implications, particularly to athletes or to anyone who wants to become very lean. Obtaining a low level of body fat is extremely difficult. It requires a large reduction in food intake, combined with a large output of calorie burning through physical activity.

Further, Metabolic Adaptations don't disappear after one has achieved his desired bodyweight loss. This is particularly true for the Fat Mass. **The Metabolic Adaptations remain.** They "command" one to eat and to refrain from physical activities. This is the deep-body's "hope" that the "patient" will be restored to his Set-Point.

These adaptations, therefore, powerfully **reduce the likelihood** of an individual's maintaining his reduced bodyweight. This is why 95-98% of people who lose weight fail to maintain the weight loss. In addition to the signals arising from the decreased Fat Mass, decreases in the Lean Body Mass send signals as well and push the body to restore its lost tissue. The forces arising from the Lean Body Mass loss don't appear to be as powerful as those arising from the Fat Mass loss.

You Must Make Adjustments When Losing Weight: What Type of Adjustments Must You Make in Response to Metabolic Adaptations from Weight Loss?

Studies show that Metabolic Adaptations occur with weight loss and calorie restriction. We must, of course, keep in mind that the strength of these adaptations depends upon two things: 1) the level of calorie restriction and 2) the initial fatness of the individual. Fatter individuals don't experience the same level of Adaptation as lean individuals. Leaner individuals experience the most powerful Metabolic Adaptations. Some of the most powerful responses occur in individuals, such as bodybuilders, undergoing attempts at weight loss.

The most detailed study of Metabolic Adaptations ever undertaken, the Minnesota Study, provides us with the opportunity of "putting-it-to-the-numbers," the all-powerful Ellis method for weight loss and weight control.

The Minnesota subjects' calorie intake before semi-starvation was 3,492 per day, a calorie intake that maintained the subjects' bodyweight at a body fat of 15%. When the study began, researchers reduced the daily calorie intake to 1,570 calories. The subjects remained on this calorie-restricted diet for the next 24-weeks. During the study, the subjects lost 25% of their initial bodyweight. Their body fat dropped to 5.3%.

At the end of the study, the men suffered from extreme depression and lethargy. The striking result was that at the end of the 24-week period, the men were no longer losing bodyweight! They were completely weight-stabilized, indicating that 1,570 calories now met their daily calorie needs. This was a reduction in calorie needs of 1,922 calories a day!

How Weight Loss (and Gain) Affect Body Composition

We need a way to express the effect of Metabolic Adaptations on calorie needs. The simplest and most effective method is to talk about how the body's need for calories decreases during weight loss. We can express Metabolic Adaptations by figuring out how many fewer calories we must eat per pound bodyweight that's lost.

To reiterate, leaner individuals need to reduce "calorie-intake-per-pound-lost" more than obese individuals because of the stronger Metabolic Adaptation signals arising from the shrunken Fat Mass. Another difference is that the signals pushing the brain to drive hunger and appetite become stronger the leaner one becomes.

These same signals also turn-on mechanisms that increase the cell's ability to "get more" out of each calorie eaten, an increase in metabolic efficiency. (Are you sure you want to be lean? It's a lot of effort, I can tell you.)

Many factors within the body determine how the body extracts the calorie's available energy. Fat people to some extent "waste" energy, dissipating it as heat. As a result, they must consume more calories to maintain their higher-than-normal bodyweight. At the other end, lean people become metabolically efficient, performing their functions by using fewer calories. So instead of using the full value of one calorie, they function adequately by consuming, say, 80%, or even less, of that one calorie. This, of course, reduces their overall calorie needs.

The metabolic **efficiency** of the lean or the metabolic **inefficiency** of the obese varies on a continuum between the two extremes of being obese or lean.

Therefore, the energy value one can extract from a calorie differs depending on body composition. Attempts to reduce bodyweight increase the body's ability to perform on fewer calories. Somewhere, in a mid-point range, all of it works as the textbook says it does.

On either side of this mid-point range, you've got to throw the rule book away.

As you move away from your Set-Point bodyweight, in either direction, up or down, a "bomb calorimeter calorie" is different from a calorie that was eaten. The "body calorie" has no less energy than the bomb calorimeter says it has. Thus, we need to use less of that calorie to perform the same work when we're lean and more of that calorie when we're fat!

Both Resting Metabolic Rate (RMR) and Physical Activity Level (PAL) are affected. In each portion of calorie burning for one who is lean, the body extracts more energy from each calorie. Or, alternatively, the body uses less energy from each calorie to perform the same functions in heavier persons.

To restate: changes in RMR are responsible for about 33% of the total decrease and changes in PAL are about 66%.

I've evaluated several studies to determine the amount of calorie decrease per pound lost. The spread of decreased calories per pound lost are from 15 calories to an extreme of 47 calories per pound lost in the Minnesota Study.

Why was there such a large adaptation in the men of the Minnesota Study? It's because they became so lean and lost so much fat that the powerful Metabolic Adaptations drove up their metabolic efficiency. As a result, they "extracted" more energy from each calorie consumed in comparison with less extreme weight loss studies. Or, alternatively, as stated above, their cells simply needed less energy to function. These men

How Weight Loss (and Gain) Affect Body Composition

maxed-out their Metabolic Adaptation machinery because of the low amount of body fat they carried.

The average reported value of decreasing calorie needs was between 20-30 calories per pound lost in the studies I evaluated. In one study of college females following a low-carbohydrate diet, researchers reported a decrease of 38 calories per pound. The college females needed to reduce their calorie intake by this amount to maintain the lighter bodyweight.

This certainly confirms the argument, that I'll present later, that the Atkins version of the low-carbohydrate diet is flawed. This is because one of Atkins' key claims is that calories don't count. The study, above, proves otherwise.

The information, above, is extremely important to your weight loss maintenance program. If you don't lower your calorie intake to meet your reduced calorie needs, I guarantee that you'll regain the weight you've lost. And it doesn't matter what type of diet you've followed in order to lose the weight. Lost weight triggers Metabolic Adaptations and there's nothing that you can do about such frustrating Adaptations other than to adjust for them by using the advanced techniques that I've developed.

The task of keeping a person's bodyweight considerably below its Set-Point by reducing calorie intake is similar to keeping body temperature and cholesterol below their natural Set-Points. These body functions are all controlled by in-born functions of control. As such, they are highly regulated and only people with an incredibly strong Willpower and the ability to tolerate physical discomfort are likely to succeed in their efforts to defeat these controls.

The use of <u>Willpower</u> to overcome <u>Biological</u> drives will always fail except in a very small percentage of individuals.

Therefore, only techniques that work in tandem with biological drives -- without calling upon Herculean displays of Moral Force and Willpower -- can possibly succeed.

Before beginning a weight loss program, you must realize that Metabolic Adaptations will ***absolutely*** occur.

When you reach your new bodyweight, you'll <u>never</u> again be able to consume the same number of calories that you consumed at the higher bodyweight if you want to maintain the lower bodyweight. If you do, you will regain the lost weight. The only way around this, of course, is to increase your activity in order to run-up your energy expenditure to your pre-weight loss level.

The following is one of the fundamental issues that you must understand. Weight control isn't easy, a fact proven by the statistic that more than 61% of the population is overweight. If it were so easy, everyone would succeed at it. The purveyors of easy weight loss programs are cheating you. If you believe that weight loss is easy, you're lying to yourself. It's going to take work, both in understanding the ***process*** of weight loss and weight control and in ***doing*** it. If you follow my plan, it will, however, become as easy as it can be!

These powerful metabolic forces operate to down-regulate many of the body's basic functions during weight loss. Conversely, the body up-regulates those same functions during weight gain.

Metabolic Adaptations add one more blockage to the attainment of a normal bodyweight -- just one more barrier to solving the weight loss and weight control equation. Since so many Americans have become

How Weight Loss (and Gain) Affect Body Composition

overweight, virtually all of us have a distorted view as to the amount of food we should stack-up on our plates. And since everyone piles their plates high, it's a natural response for each of us to do the same thing. This, of course, becomes a vicious cycle, contributing to the ever-growing obesity problem.

The purpose of reduced calorie burning is to avoid further losses of fat which, in survival terms, protects the body. The power of this calorie-reducing drive is a function of the size of the fat stores. This is good for survival but bad for an individual wanting to maintain their weight loss after dieting.

After bodyweight reduction, the body's normal dynamisms try to return the individual to a newly-established, higher Fat Mass Set-Point. The body forgets the original in-born memory. This, of course, becomes another blockage to success that must be accounted for in weight loss maintenance. Individuals will have to think about, understand, and use controls to overcome these Biological drives. These techniques are embodied in the concept of Behavior Modification, meaning that one must be **aware** of the actions they can use to avoid relapse. I'll discuss the key methods within the technique of Behavior Modification later.

At the other extreme of deviation from the normal Set-Point are individuals, such as athletes, who become very lean. Bodybuilders are an excellent example. They attain body fat percent levels of between 4-6% at competition time. The amount of effort required to attain this level of fat loss is extraordinary, as I know, having achieved similar levels myself. Even less!

During my own years of experimentation, I experienced the Metabolic Adaptations described above at both extremes: during overfeeding and underfeeding. It's only recently, however, that I've come to understand the mechanisms underlying the changes that occurred in me during these two different experiments.

When I attained my highest bodyweight of 265 pounds, I found it impossible to maintain it. The forces driving me back toward my Set-Point were extremely powerful. I *forced* myself to consume the 10,000 calories a day required to attain that bodyweight. I had no appetite, I was nauseous, and had no interest in food.

At the lowest bodyweight that I'd attained, 165 pounds, the forces' powerful drive created tremendous suffering. I was starving, constantly wanting to eat, depressed, lethargic, and exhausted. It was impossible to maintain that bodyweight. I now understand why I would always gravitate either upward, or downward, between 215-220 pounds. That was, and is, my Set-Point.

What is the Mechanism Behind "Post-Starvation Obesity?"

Almost everyone who's ever completed a weight loss program has suffered from this same problem of post-starvation obesity. Recent re-evaluations of the Minnesota Study show that the depleted Fat Mass exerts a very powerful stimulus on the brain's feeding centers that drives both hunger and appetite leading to an extreme hyperphagia (ravenous intake of food, overeating).

Sound familiar? The magnitude of overeating arises from the extent of depletion of both the Fat Mass and Lean Body Mass. The degree of Fat Mass loss, however, is the stronger determinant of the two in driving overeating.

The overeating response is also dictated by both the fat-stores memory and the Lean Body Mass-stores memory. The *functional* importance of this increase in

How Weight Loss (and Gain) Affect Body Composition

hunger and appetite is that it accelerates the re-building of both Fat Mass and Lean Body Mass.

The strongest determinant of Metabolic Adaptations, as I've shown, is a signal arising from the depleted Fat Mass and this Fat Mass signal is the driving force behind bodyweight recovery. Its origin is most profoundly the "need" to accelerate the re-building of the fat stores.

This all leads, needless to say, to a **disproportionate** rate of fat recovery relative to Lean Body Mass recovery. First, the Fat Mass reaches 100% of the body's original Fat Mass. This is, of course, the level the body possessed just-prior to the start of calorie restriction. At this point, however, Lean Body Mass recovery lags behind, well below its 100% level.

The overeating continues, however, until the Lean Body Mass reaches 100% of the amount possessed by the subject previous to food restriction. Unfortunately, by this time, the Fat Mass has risen to about 150% of its original amount.

At the completion of tissue recovery, finally, overeating slows. Gradually, over time, the body's in-born controls automatically lower food intake. One begins, then, to return to his normal bodyweight Set-Point.

Unfortunately, many people fail to adapt, never reducing their overeating and remain at a higher bodyweight.

You must have an understanding of these adaptive responses to food restriction and bodyweight loss which is essential in designing and using effective strategies to **Biologically** control this expected, automatic occurrence.

Most nutritional counselors and medical personnel recommend a low-fat diet. This diet, though, is directly responsible for driving food into the Fat Mass because it stimulates fat-making enzymes (I'll discuss this in detail in the following chapters).

These fat-making enzymes convert carbohydrates into body fat. By definition, low-fat diets are also high in carbohydrates. These carbohydrates, via fat-making enzymes, stimulate a process that converts them into saturated human fat and the body subsequently stores this "fat-made-from-carbohydrate" within the Fat Mass.

Consumption of a low-carbohydrate diet, conversely, accelerates the growth of the Lean Body Mass while minimizing the repletion of the Fat Mass. ***In this way, we reverse the normal order of events and work synergistically with nature instead of fighting her.***

We don't fully remove the Metabolic Adaptation signals arising from the depleted Fat Mass but we do remove some of the other signals that stimulate hunger and appetite both of which drive overeating.

These responses characterize the typical Metabolic Adaptations experienced by everybody undergoing food restriction and the only way to avoid these adaptations is to use the methods that I'll teach you. You will use these methods along with the requisite cognitive controls embodied within Behavior Modification.

● ●

I described in an earlier chapter how the calorie content of a food is determined. The food is placed in an oven called a bomb calorimeter and burned until it's reduced to ashes. A water jacket, surrounding the oven, accumulates an amount of heat equivalent to the calorie content (heat content) of the food under study.

How Weight Loss (and Gain) Affect Body Composition

We've now gained a fascinating insight as a result of our exploration of Metabolic Adaptations. The calorie content of a food, measured by bomb calorimetry -- and the representation of that "bomb calorimeter calorie content of a food" in charts and on food packaging -- is very different from what happens to that calorie when it enters the body.

In other words, the calorie value of a food, once we eat it, is a very different <u>beast</u> from the calorie content of the food that we read about in books and calculate for placing on labels.

As you move away from your Set-Point bodyweight, in either direction, up or down, a "bomb calorimeter calorie" is different from a calorie that has entered the body. The "body calorie" has no less energy than the bomb calorimeter says it has. When we become lean we need to use less of that calorie to perform the same work. When we become fat we need to use more of that calorie!

When do Metabolic Adaptations really become strong? We have very little data because the research in this area is small. One study shows that they kick-in strongly when you've lost about 10% of your bodyweight.

But, remember, your initial Fat Mass is a determining factor. The leaner you become, the harder it is to lose because the body becomes metabolically efficient, functioning effectively by extracting less energy from each calorie.

And when is a "bomb calorimeter calorie" the same as an "eaten calorie?" My guess is that it's the same when one is close to his Set-Point bodyweight. And what is that? It is, probably, the bodyweight at which one's Body Mass Index (BMI) is between 21-23. (Remember, we discussed this calculation in an earlier chapter. It's a calculation that you should have, by now, determined.)

A BMI of 20 is about equal to 12% body fat in males and 22% in females; a BMI of 25 is about 22% fat in males and 30% fat in females. Therefore, the BMI range of 20-25 is the normal human mid-point range, and, most likely, most metabolic actions are of the textbook variety when you're in this range.

The average male fat percent is estimated at 15%, and the average female fat percent is 24%. My fat percent at 215-220 pounds is about 15%. A BMI of 22 and a fat percent of 15% in males and of 24% in females are most likely the Set-Point ranges for humans. When one is in this Set-Point range, he or she doesn't have to fight Metabolic Adaptations.

Calculating his BMI won't work for an athlete because he inflates his Lean Body Mass because he builds muscle beyond the normal, predictable textbook relationship that exists between Lean Body Mass and Height, as I've described previously. Therefore, his BMI will always be in the overweight range, even though he may be very lean.

Because of his fat-stores memory, an obese individual, reducing from a BMI of, say, 35 to one of 24 (the normal range), may experience Metabolic Adaptations because he distorted his normal metabolic ranges and his "memory" of them by becoming obese.

The use of my advanced methods is critical to the obese person who attempts to reduce down to a normal bodyweight. These methods help him quash the powerful drives of all the calorie-sparing mechanisms driving his body to use fewer calories.

As one moves lower or higher relative to the 20-25 BMI range, the activity of Metabolic Adaptations becomes stronger. It takes a great deal of effort to push bodyweight lower.

How Weight Loss (and Gain) Affect Body Composition

It's easier, though, to push BMI (bodyweight) higher, rather than lower because gaining weight requires a combination of eating more food and performing less physical activity.

Many people are able to easily do both. The ease of becoming obese, rather than being lean, is obvious since so many people are overweight, rather than lean.

Anyone working in weight control has had plenty of experience in setting up a straight-line weight loss program for a client. After he loses 10 pounds, he reports that he's no longer losing. We sit down and check all of the numbers and reassure him that, if he's following the program, he should lose weight. We then berate him and accuse him of lying about following the program. He then squeals in disbelief that we don't believe him, and the whole situation turns ugly.

Clearly, there are many situations in which clients aren't following the programs. But just as clearly, there are clients who are following their programs, but it's no longer working. This is why so many say the calorie theory is wrong, such as Dr. Atkins.

This is because it can't work any longer. These are the clients who have metabolically adapted. The programs must be **adjusted** to meet these changes in order for them continue losing.

This information is empowering because it solves one of the major problems in weight loss and weight control. So remember, a calorie in a bomb calorimeter is often not the same as a calorie that has entered the body. And the variability in the use of the calorie's energy depends upon:

1) the body's placement on its body composition continuum

2) and on the degree that it has deviated from its Set-Point!

••••••••••••••••••••••••••

It's always easier, **Biologically**, to lose weight when starting at a higher initial fat content. Unfortunately, the things that led to the overweight condition in the first place may make it **psychologically** more difficult to lose weight because these psychological characteristics are so difficult to overcome. But, as we've seen, the leaner you become, the more difficult it is to continue to lose fat.

Major changes in the body's tissues evoke powerful signals arising from the tissue changes. These, in turn, stimulate alterations in the genes, the enzyme systems, the hormonal system, and the nervous system. These changes have dramatic effects on the brain, the organs, and, ultimately, on every part of the body. They affect behavior related to eating and moving, the two sides of the Energy Balance Equation.

By following my program, you'll never miss the mark again. You'll be in **complete control**, knowing exactly what steps to take in order to achieve your goals.

But I'll guarantee you that, no matter what your goal -- whether it's reducing from 300 pounds to 250 pounds, or reducing from 10% body fat to 5% body fat -- my program has the techniques to help achieve those goals.

We're now going to delve into the specific dietary and exercise programs that, when conscientiously practiced, will help you achieve your goals. The dietary information affects the Energy-In (calories eaten) part of the Energy Balance Equation. The exercise and physical activity information affects the Energy-Out (calories burned) part of that Equation.

Chapter 7

The Power of Eating the Right Type of Food

We're now ready to dive into techniques to control the Law of Nature: the Energy Balance Equation. Scientists, doctors, nutritionists, and even people without degrees in dietetics or nutrition have developed weight loss programs and the number of weight loss programs is beyond belief. However, only one guiding fact exists: maintaining proper bodyweight is a function of the Energy Balance Equation.

There's a flaw in any method that doesn't accept and embrace this fact. There's no secret or mystery about weight control. We know, now, all that we need to know to solve this problem. However, secrets do exist about how to **optimize** the Energy Balance Equation. These secrets are hidden in the complicated writings characteristic of the scientific literature. I had to squeeze them from the entangled research web where these secrets were often lost in misinterpretations of data.

The Energy Balance Equation has two parts, Energy-In and Energy-Out. It's the balancing, or the unbalancing, between the two sides that determines bodyweight. In the following chapters, I'll describe how food choices affect the Energy-In side of the Equation. In later chapters, I'll describe how physical activity affects the Energy-Out side.

I've already described that calorie balance is the most important factor in bodyweight regulation.

First, however, before detailing diet composition, I want to let you in on a secret, a little-known fact that's important to bodyweight and body composition control. Later, I'll teach you the biochemical control systems that

The Power of Eating the Right Type of Food

determine what happens to food once it's eaten. Then I'll provide the details about this secret. This secret is critically important and **is the underlying mechanism determining your drive to eat.**

Everyone assumes that the number of calories that **goes into the mouth** is the same number of calories **available to be burned.** This common belief, however, isn't true.

The calories from food consumed have two fates: they are burned for energy or stored as an energy reserve, primarily in fat tissue. This distribution of fuel is termed energy-partitioning. The body, therefore, **actually monitors the food that's burned; it doesn't monitor the calories that go into the mouth**!

If the food that you eat is locked in storage in fat tissue, it's not available to be burned. It becomes available only when conditions change allowing the fat cell to release its stored supply of fat.

When the food is stored in fat tissue, it's as if you hadn't eaten the food in the first place. Unfortunately, you did eat it and now, it's part of your fat stores. Energy-partitioning depends primarily on the type of food that one eats: carbohydrates, proteins, or fats. And, of the three, it's the carbohydrates that drive the energy-partitioning of fuel into the fat stores. The body converts a portion of the carbohydrate into fat storage! Proteins and fats, in the absence of carbohydrates, don't drive energy-partitioning of fuel into the fat stores.

To control the Energy-In portion of the Energy Balance Equation, we must use techniques that control **appetite** and **hunger.** Applying methods that control appetite Biologically are the best methods. Using Willpower is the worst method to succeed in controlling food intake. To control food intake we must recruit

Biology as an ally. Remember, using Willpower is a weak second-best to using Biological controls.

Using Willpower is like trying to hold your breath. You can try and you'll last a minute or two. Then, Biological control systems will force you to gasp for air. Attempting to use Willpower to control food intake has the same outcome. The only difference is time. The body's Biology expresses itself quickly in the control of breathing. You can only stop breathing for a minute or two. Controlling the drive to eat is easier than breath holding. You can reduce food intake to the point of hunger. And, you can "Willpower yourself" through hunger control for a while. Without doubt, though, within several weeks, or at most several months, however, hunger will overpower you. You'll gasp for food. Then, you'll eat voraciously, regaining all the weight you lost.

How We Define Diet Composition

Foods have varying proportions of carbohydrates, fats, and proteins. These are called the macronutrients. Vitamins and minerals are called micronutrients. Carbohydrates and fats serve primarily as sources of fuel. Proteins serve to maintain the structural parts of the body. The body can convert protein to carbohydrate. When it does so, the body uses protein for energy.

It's clear, then, that the composition of your diet is an important issue. Diet composition influences bodyweight and body composition. A spirited debate has arisen over this issue of diet composition over the last several decades because of the growing interest in the low-carbohydrate diet. Researchers have, for many years, explored the influence of diet composition on changes in bodyweight and body composition. It seems 'logical' that the fat you eat becomes the fat on your body. Most people, therefore, avoid fat consumption because they

The Power of Eating the Right Type of Food

believe that "fat-goes-to-fat."

Diet composition is the percent of each of the three energy foods -- protein, carbohydrates, and fat -- in the diet. Over the years, scientists have tried varying all three.

For simplicity though, there are three primary variations of diet composition: the low-fat diet, the low-carbohydrate diet, and the mixed diet. A low-fat diet is 15-30% of the daily calorie intake as fat. A low-carbohydrate diet, however, has a different definition depending on the designator. It shouldn't, but it does.

Scientists usually consider a low-carbohydrate diet one in which 45-50% of its calories is carbohydrate. Proponents of the low-carbohydrate diet believe that this diet should contain between 60-80 **grams** of carbohydrate per day. If one consumed 2,500 calories per day, 80 grams yields 13% of the calories as carbohydrate.

The mixed diet is typical of what most people consume. It's composed of about 15%-protein, 40%-fat, and 45%-carbohydrate. Scientists call this diet the "super-market" or the "cafeteria" diet. It's well known that this type of diet leads to overweight and obesity, a fact beyond dispute, a fact that even I agree with.

Scientists refer to the super-market diet as a high-fat diet. Unfortunately, they have left out another key term for this diet and that is that this diet is also a high-carbohydrate diet. Therefore, it is both high-fat **and** high-carbohydrate. Misstating the true link between the carbohydrate and fat content in the super-market diet has produced an enormous amount of confusion. It has confused both scientists and the public.

Unraveling the Diet Composition Mystery

Unraveling the complex and twisted story of diet composition has been the roller coaster ride of my life. There have been more twists and turns than I could ever have imagined when I began my studies. There are endless opinions about the effects of diet composition on bodyweight and body composition. This subject is complex.

An omission, such as the one I described above, leads to the publication of hundreds, even thousands, of research papers that all make the same omission. This, of course, further clouds the issue. Mining the truth has been an arduous task, one requiring years of work.

The majority of nutritional scientists have bought into the idea that fat is bad. Fat is the villain responsible for cancer, heart disease, diabetes, and obesity. These scientists continue to publish research papers supporting the edifice they've created. They serve on international committees. They develop large groups of sympathetic colleagues, working together in supporting the growing dogma. In the bibliographies at the end of their research papers, they list only research that supports their position. They rarely list research conflicting with their ideas. Often, they don't even know that conflicting research exists.

My Conversion

As a teenager and during my early 20's, I had consumed a high-protein, low-carbohydrate diet by happenstance. I had no sense about what I was doing. I knew that I wanted to consume lots of grams of protein to build my muscles. By 1990, I had been through my vegetarian phase. That was the most extreme form of low-fat eating possible (except for fasting). In the 1980's, armed with my advanced measuring techniques, I began

The Power of Eating the Right Type of Food

my high-carbohydrate, low-fat diet. I began a systematic program of measuring the changes occurring in my body. Both of these eating regimens, vegetarianism and complex carbohydrate, turned out to be failures. Neither helped me to reach my goal of more muscle mass and less fat.

Late in the 1980's, I decided to pursue, again, the low-carbohydrate diet. I decided to follow the Atkins version of the low-carbohydrate diet. I promptly gained 5 pounds. I realized, then, that there were major limitations to his version of the low-carbohydrate regimen.

During the pursuit of my Ph. D. degree, I'd become familiar with the biochemistry of fuel metabolism and its regulation. I'd come to understand that muscles and organs **preferred** to burn fat as their primary fuel (Atkins doesn't even know this fact). The majority of scientists, and the public, believe that these tissues prefer to burn carbohydrate.

My statement that fat is the primary fuel will turn a lot of heads, even those of scientists. I described the research showing that fat is the primary fuel for muscles and organs in the introduction to my Ph. D. thesis. Since I'm sure you won't be reading it, I want to quote from the classic biochemistry textbook, Lehninger's <u>Principles of Biochemistry</u>. "In resting muscle the primary fuels are free fatty acids from adipose tissue and ketone bodies from the liver. The use of blood glucose and muscle glycogen as **emergency** (emphasis mine) fuels for muscular activity is greatly enhanced by the secretion of epinephrine, which stimulates the formation of blood glucose from glycogen in the liver and the breakdown of glycogen in muscle tissue." I want to make it clear that I am right about the muscles and organs preferring fat as their primary source of fuel because some other Ph. D. will surely dispute me. But I'm right and he's wrong.

Because I knew the fact that muscles prefer to burn fat, it made sense to continue studying the low-carbohydrate diet. I continued to follow a low-carbohydrate diet in spite of my failure with Atkins' version. I wanted to understand how the low-carbohydrate diet worked. I figured that when I understood how it worked I'd develop an effective version of my own. Then, I could meet my goals.

There's a relationship between what goes on at the cellular level and the end result of that cellular activity. The end result of the activity in the cells reflects itself by changes at the whole body level. There are changes, for instance, in the amount of muscle tissue and fat tissue contained in the body. I understood that the low-carbohydrate diet increased muscle tissue and decreased fat tissue. This made sense because I knew that the low-carbohydrate diet pushed fuel into the active tissues, the organs and muscles, and stimulated the release of fat from fat cells. This was a biochemical fact. I did not yet fully understand, however, the mechanisms involved.

I began, at that juncture, a very detailed study about the relationship between the controls related to the body's handling of carbohydrates and its handling of fats. I studied the biochemical pathways within the **cell** that controlled fuel use and then I studied the changes in the **whole body** in response to this cellular activity. Although the Atkins' low-carbohydrate version failed often, I knew that was because of a quirk in it. It wasn't because of the low-carbohydrate diet, itself. I spent endless hours in the medical library, collecting hundreds of papers about diet composition, desperately trying to unravel the conflicting information.

Many publications, of course, dealt with the interactions between carbohydrates and fats. As a graduate student, I'd developed the habit of investigating the history of the subjects I explored. This technique would prove invaluable in my coming to understand present-day nutritional theories.

Carbohydrate-to-Fat Conversion

Very quickly, my research efforts uncovered studies about the relationship between carbohydrate and fat feeding. Scientists had long wondered whether fat could form from non-fat sources. In fact, the first experimental proof of carbohydrate-to-fat conversion was presented in 1852. Further experiments, in 1901, suggested that rapid fat formation occurred from eating carbohydrates. Researchers showed that when animals were fed a grain diet they rapidly converted carbohydrate into body fat. It was well understood, by the 1960's, that low-fat, high-carbohydrate diets led to a rapid conversion of carbohydrate-to-fat. The name of this biochemical process is lipogenesis -- <u>lipo</u> meaning fat, <u>genesis</u> meaning formation -- fat formation from carbohydrate.

An early, and very important finding, was detailed in a 1950 study published in the *Journal of Biological Chemistry*. This study showed that rats fed a 100%-carbohydrate diet rapidly converted carbohydrate into fat in their livers. In this study, the rats were underfed, consuming fewer calories than needed to meet their energy needs. They lost weight, and this should have shifted their metabolism with fuel directed to the active tissues: fat storage from food should have shut down. But instead, the livers were transformed into fat-making factories under the influence of the high-carbohydrate diet!

At this time, in 1990, I hadn't yet embraced the Energy Balance Equation. I didn't understand its total importance. I did understand, however, that, if calories were under-consumed, weight would be lost because energy needs aren't being met and the body consumes its stored fuel. This calorie deficiency drives fuel into the active tissues. A source of this fuel is fat stored in adipose tissue.

But, surprisingly, the 100%-carbohydrate diet actually overrode this expected response and the liver actually turned-on its fat-making capacity, converting carbohydrate into stored fat.

The opening sentences of the 1950 publication state, "That carbohydrate utilization depends upon an animal's previous nutritional state has long been recognized and is supported by an overwhelming amount of evidence. Thus glucose (blood sugar) utilization is depressed in the fasted animal and in the animal fed a diet containing little or no carbohydrate."

Other findings supported this idea, "Generally, dietary carbohydrates increase liver lipogenesis (fat-making from carbohydrate) and the activities of enzymes related to lipogenesis, whereas dietary fats or starvation have the opposite effect."

In 1955, researchers from Jefferson Medical College, Philadelphia, wanted to see if the liver's capacity for lipogenesis (fat-making) was different from that of adipose tissue. Their conclusions were, "Feeding a high-carbohydrate diet stimulated lipogenesis in adipose (fat tissue), which considerably exceeded that found in the liver. The assumption that adipose tissue is the main site of lipogenesis is supported by the observation of an unimpaired lipogenesis in animals without livers." And, "The rate of lipogenesis from available carbohydrates seems to be regulated by the carbohydrate content of the diet." Finally, "Fasting or feeding a high-fat diet abolished lipogenesis in adipose tissue."

Abolished. Wow! Stopped it altogether. A high-fat diet stops fat making, and a high-carbohydrate diet turns fat making on. Think about **this** the next time you read the experts' recommendations about the healthfulness of the high-carbohydrate diet.

I now had the evidence convincing me that high-carbohydrate feeding makes one fat. How fat one becomes depends on calorie balance. This evidence also showed that high-fat/low-carbohydrate feeding doesn't make one fat as long as calorie intake doesn't exceed calorie burning. There was one problem with this research. The adipose tissue and livers had been cut out of these animals. The effects of carbohydrate feeding had been isolated from the whole animal. People might argue that carbohydrate-to-fat conversion doesn't occur in whole living organisms but occurs only in the isolated cell fragments.

Fortunately, it didn't take long to find the answer as to whether diet composition affected body composition. I found a paper, published in 1990, that addressed this issue. It was a head-to-head comparison of the two different diets. One group of rats ate a high-carbohydrate/low-fat diet (63%-carbohydrate/13%-fat). The other group ate a high-fat/low-carbohydrate diet (63%-fat/13%-carbohydrate). Both groups ate this way for 44 days.

It was beyond argument that these two different diets led to dramatic differences in body composition. The high-fat/low-carbohydrate fed rats weighed only 252 grams, compared with 282 grams for the high-carbohydrate/low-fat fed animals. Most striking was the difference in body fat. The high-fat/low-carbohydrate rats had only 22 grams of body fat (9% body fat). The high-carbohydrate/low-fat fed group had a whopping 65 grams of body fat (23% fat).

This was the perfect complementary research to the studies done 40 years earlier. It powerfully confirmed that high-carbohydrate eating leads to its own conversion to body fat. The clincher was this. The rat bodies on the high-fat/low-carbohydrate diet contained more protein (muscles and organs).

Now, let's think about these studies, above, for a moment. The finding that carbohydrate converts to fat implies that one should eat few carbohydrates. Even more striking is the fact that carbohydrate converts to fat during a calorie deficiency! This implies that diet composition somehow affects the Energy Balance Equation.

This effect is independent of Energy-In and Energy-Out.

Carbohydrate that's converted to fat is stored. Those calories are no longer available to the active tissues! **This is the essence of energy-partitioning.** Eating a calorie doesn't mean that that calorie remains available to the active tissues as fuel.

This is a mind-numbing revelation. This surely adds a new dimension to the calorie tables, doesn't it?

Energy-partitioning and Metabolic Adaptations don't nullify the Energy Balance Equation. They do, however, make an impact upon it. We must account for them when using the Energy Balance Equation for weight loss and weight control purposes.

My growing file of research papers was convincing me that high-carbohydrate diets contributed to increases in body fat. These increases occurred **at the same time as** decreases in muscle tissue. These changes occurred even during times of calorie deficiency. The research papers demonstrated that the mechanism behind these changes was the conversion of carbohydrate to fat.

The fact was, however, that carbohydrate stimulated its own conversion to fat. Certainly, no one knows why this occurs. It's just an evolutionary fact. I believe the reason behind it is that during man's evolution little carbohydrate was available as a food source. The body's metabolic machinery developed as a result of consuming mostly meat and fat from animals. That was the primary diet of early humans. Therefore, the body's machinery didn't tolerate carbohydrates very well. And for whatever reason, the body developed a biochemical process to store carbohydrates as fat. We'll never know the real reason why the body did this. But, what we do know is that this is precisely what it does: converts carbohydrate into fat.

There's overwhelming scientific confirmation of these conversions of carbohydrate to body fat, and they date back more than 140 years.

Chapter 8

Why Low-Fat Diets Don't Work

Low-fat dieting is all the rage today. You can't pick up a magazine or a newspaper, look at a TV show, or talk to anyone without hearing about the value of low-fat dieting. Proponents say that a low-fat diet helps you lose weight. Just as important, they say that it's "heart-healthy" too. The low-fat diet is based upon the belief that fat makes you fat. Further, many people believe that the low-fat diet satisfies the appetite: that one automatically eats fewer calories by eating low-fat foods. In this way, one avoids the drudgery of counting calories. By the use of such "automatic" controls, it's believed, the dieter reduces food intake effortlessly.

If, dear reader, you're following a low-fat diet, I'm sorry to disappoint you because there's no proof that low-fat dieting works to control weight and food intake. In fact, most scientific studies prove that the change in diet composition to a low-fat diet makes little, if any, difference in weight control.

This chapter was deleted from Ultimate Diet Secrets Lite. But if you want it, I provide it as a FREE e-chapter in the Adobe PDF format. Just go to my web site at www.ultimatedietsecrets.com. For those of you without internet access I will provide in the following several pages the most critical elements of this chapter to show you why low-fat eating was such an abysmal failure.

In 1992, the National Institutes of Health (NIH) made a Consensus Conference Statement for Methods for Voluntary Weight Loss and Control: "There is evidence that altering the proportion of the calories in the diet from fat, carbohydrate, and protein can have a limited effect on weight loss. However, the effects appear to be quite small in comparison with the direct effect of caloric restriction."

In spite of the NIH statement, the most popular and most recommended weight control diet is the low-fat, high complex carbohydrate diet. Most experts also recommend this diet for good health and disease prevention. These experts believe that low-fat foods control weight and that low-fat eating improves health at the same time.

The current diet recommendations include cutting fat to 30% or less of daily calories and saturated fat to less than 10%. Protein percentages are usually the same in all diet recommendations, about 12-16% of daily calories. Therefore, carbohydrates, with the emphasis on complex carbohydrates, make up about 55% of daily calories. Experts encourage us to eat this so-called "balanced diet."

Most health organizations recommend this diet too. The most aggressive groups (groups that hate fat), however, believe that we should cut fat to 20% or even to 10% of daily calories. Only time will tell whether these beliefs are accepted. These recommendations, it's clear, push the nation's dietary direction towards vegetarianism.

Evidence About Low-fat Diets and Weight Loss

Let's look at some of the evidence about the effects of low-fat diets on weight control. Remember, any diet bases its success, if any, on the Energy Balance Equation. Every scientist agrees with this. Additional benefits, such as faster weight loss or increases in muscle tissue, may arise from following a plan that varies diet composition. These changes will be minor in effect, however, compared with changing how much one eats and how much one burns.

As we've seen, the fact is that it's carbohydrates that go directly to the fat cells. Ingesting fat, in the absence of carbohydrate, shuttles fuel into the active tissues for burning.

Group	Baseline cals	1-year cals	1-year difference in weight	2-year cals	2-year total difference in weight
Control	1,713	1,572		1,606	
Low-Fat	1,736	1,297	– 5.7 lbs.	1,342	– 4.0 lbs.

In a low-fat study (see the table above) subjects lost a total of 4 pounds following the low-fat diet for two years, an abysmal response. The researchers had combined the low-fat diet with extensive educational programs. The education programs discussed the "how-to" of losing and controlling bodyweight. The researchers concluded that their statistical analysis had proved that a low percent of energy eaten as fat had a <u>strong</u> association with weight loss.

They made this statement even though the **bodyweights of the two groups were not statistically different.** This result -- no difference in bodyweight -- does not support their conclusion. They cannot legitimately claim that the number of calories consumed as fat is a strong predictor of bodyweight gain or loss.

Even using my less precise not-so-scientific concept, of practical significance, it's obvious that low-fat was not a strong predictor of weight loss. Nevertheless, this is how it goes in research paper after research paper. No wonder it took me more than 40 years to figure it out.

With statistical analysis, one can test to see which factors contribute to the changes observed. We can use a more "understandable" analysis based on a 100% scale. In the study, above, using this type of analysis, percent

Why Low-Fat Diets Don't Work

of calories as fat contributed only 11% to the weight gain. I'd be surprised if 11% convinced you that percent of fat calories was a <u>strong</u> predictor of weight gain. This statement is similar to the misleading statements made by the cholesterol and heart disease researchers.

The researchers performed this analysis only at the end of the first year because, during the second year, the subjects began to regain weight. After 2-years of a near-starvation diet, averaging about 1,300 calories a day, the subjects lost about 4 pounds. Whoopee! That's something to write home about? A four pound weight loss is nothing to brag about after so much training, nutritional instruction, and yes, famine-like intake of calories.

Neither group ate many calories to begin with. In addition, this study was "confounded" meaning that the researchers used multiple treatments in the experiment. The treatment group used 1) a low-fat diet, 2) nutrition training, 3) behavioral change, and 4) self-monitoring tools.

In the study, above, which treatment led to the decrease in the calories the subjects ate? Which treatment led to the loss in weight? Moreover, even if we could find out which treatment led to the observed differences, those differences were meager at best. They weren't even statistically significant.

One could easily drop 4 pounds during 4 months. There's no need to change one's diet, no need to take classes in nutrition education, and no need for a counselor to encourage one to stick with the program. Just walk about 1 mile each day!

Low-fat Mania Overtakes the Country

If the above facts don't convince you as to the ineffectiveness of low-fat dieting, then go ahead, eat low-fat.

In 2001, I performed a quasi-scientific poll about people's beliefs as to the how-to of controlling bodyweight. I asked: "Which one of the following two factors is the more important in weight control: 1) the total number of calories that one eats in a day or 2) the total amount of fat that one eats in a day?"

I was stunned when 7 out of 10 people chose the latter, the total amount of fat eaten. They believed that total fat consumption was the most important factor in weight control. This idea has become a part of the nations' collective consciousness. It pervades our thinking, our conversations, and our writing. It is, however, dead wrong.

The tacit acceptance of the low-fat diet as a panacea for preventing weight gain or for bodyweight control **has no basis in science**. Yet, most people believe it and believe that by cutting down on fat intake, they will lose fat and control their bodyweight. It's not true.

Many scientific studies have explored the value of fats versus carbohydrates in satisfying appetite. There's been a lot of emphasis on the low-fat diet. There have also been many studies of the low-carbohydrate diet and its ability to satisfy appetite. But the low-fat supporters never cite these studies in their research papers. There are two different nutritional factions: the low-fat lovers and the low-carbohydrate lovers. The low-carbohydrate lovers, far fewer in number than the low-fat lovers, lower carbohydrates enough in their studies to see the effects of a true low-carbohydrate diet.

Why Low-Fat Diets Don't Work

The low-fat lovers use a model of what they call a low-carbohydrate diet compared with the low-fat diet. But it's never low enough in carbohydrate to register as a true low-carbohydrate diet. Nonetheless, they haven't uncovered any significant differences between fat's and carbohydrate's ability to satisfy hunger. So, even though they use a watered-down version of the low-carbohydrate diet it still satisfies hunger as well as their much beloved low-fat diet. This must really aggravate them.

My position, however, is that the **primary** reason for the rapid increases in bodyweight is not a dietary cause, but a cause arising from decreases in physical activity.

Unfortunately, those recommending this diet are unaware that high-carbohydrate diets cause the conversion of carbohydrate into fat which is, of course, at the expense of muscle tissue.

"But Fat Has Twice as Many Calories per Gram vs. Carbohydrate. Eat Fat, and You Eat Two Times More Calories," say the Low-fat Proponents

One of the main arguments raised by supporters of low-fat dieting is that fat has 9 calories per gram, and carbohydrate, only 4 calories per gram. In this argument, fat has more than twice as many calories per gram compared with carbohydrate. They're right, of course.

They claim that, if you eat 50 grams of fat, you put 450 calories into your mouth. If you eat 50 grams of carbohydrate, you eat only 200 calories. They're right about this too.

So their theory is this: we can substitute low-fat, low-energy density foods (high-carbohydrate) for high-fat. This substitution is a diet aid because eating 50 grams of carbohydrate, instead of 50 grams of fat, lowers calorie intake by 250 calories.

The weakness of this argument is the **assumption** that you'll eat the same number of **grams** of both fat and carbohydrate. Most experimental studies show that, if one eats less carbohydrate, he'll eat more fat and conversely, if one eats less fat, he eats more carbohydrates to meet calorie needs. He eats for calories, not for grams of food. (The argument, above, has one major weakness that its supporters aren't aware of: if one cuts carbohydrates to a certain threshold, he'll eat fewer calories. I'll tell you more about this in the next chapter).

One eats for calories that are burned, not for <u>grams</u> of food.

In summary, there's no proof that low-fat dieting is more effective for weight control than eating whatever type of food one wants. Controlling calorie intake is most important. One can eat less or move more. No matter how you cut the cards, it's energy balance that controls.

Chapter 9

The Complete Scoop on the Low-Carbohydrate Diet

Let me state it here and now. I don't want any confusion about this. The low-carbohydrate diet is effective for two reasons, and two reasons only:

1) **it reduces food intake, and**
2) **it's the best dietary method to reduce body fat and increase muscle mass. Period. No more to it.**

Don't expect anything more. There's no magic beyond these effects. These are good enough, magic indeed in their power. A low-carbohydrate diet is a **part** of the total weight loss and weight control equation but it **serves under** the Energy Balance Equation, which rules supremely.

Interest is growing, however, in weight control through the mechanisms of the low-carbohydrate diet. I don't want the same misconceptions mistreating the low-carbohydrate diet that blessed the low-fat diet: I don't want, that is, people to believe that low-carbohydrate diets are more powerful than the Energy Balance Equation. Just as low-fat eating is not a free-for-all for eating, low-carbohydrate eating isn't a license to eat as much food as you want either. Many would have you believe that it's just such a license for dietary excess (Dr. Atkins and Suzanne Somers). It isn't.

History of the Low-Carbohydrate Diet

Low-carbohydrate diets have a long history, dating back to 1856 in England. In 1953, Dr. A. W. Pennington introduced the diet to the executives of the Dupont Company in Wilmington, Delaware. Over the years, it has cropped-up in the Stillman Diet, in <u>The Diet Revolution</u> of Dr. Atkins, and in several others. Millions of people have had success with the carbohydrate-restricted diet.

Many supporters of the diet, however, have anointed it with magical properties with the first proposals coming from Dr. Pennington. This was, later, particularly true of Dr. Atkins who adopted the "metabolic magic" proclamations and still does so to this day, in 2002.

In 1960, Dr. John Yudkin proved beyond any doubt ***that any effective weight loss changes came from the reduction in calories***. People simply ate fewer calories when their diet was low in carbohydrates. That was the magic: it was just easier for people to eat less, supporting, of course, my emphasis on the Energy Balance Equation.

The Ketone Story

Low-carbohydrate diets are also called Ketogenic diets because ketone levels increase in the blood and urine (for a little while) of dieters eating few carbohydrates. Ketones arise from the fatty acid molecules released by fat cells.

The storage form of fat in the adipose tissue is as a triglyceride, whose molecule looks like the letter E. The vertical line of the letter E is the backbone, called the glycerol part of the triglyceride molecule. The three horizontal lines represent the long chain fatty acids. For simplicity, each horizontal line, each long chain fatty acid, is made of 18 carbon atoms connected to one another, as in the drawing below.

C-C-C-C-C-C-C-C-C-C-C-C-C-C-C-C-C-C
|
C-C-C-C-C-C-C-C-C-C-C-C-C-C-C-C-C-C
|
C-C-C-C-C-C-C-C-C-C-C-C-C-C-C-C-C-C
  1   18

    The three 18-carbon chains split from the glycerol backbone, one at a time. The tri- (3-chain) glyceride becomes a di- (2-chain) glyceride, then a mono (1-chain) glyceride as each 18-carbon chain splits off. Then, the 18-carbon chains leave the adipose cell and flow into the blood. Once in the blood, they connect to and are transported by a blood protein called albumin.

C-C-C-C-C-C-C-C-C-C-C-C-C-C-C-C-C-C
|
C-C-C-C-C-C-C-C-C-C-C-C-C-C-C-C-C-C
|
C-an 18 carbon chain splits (see below):

    Now, when they leave the fat cell and enter the blood, the 18-carbon chains are called ***free fatty acids***:

C-C-C-C-C-C-C-C-C-C-C-C-C-C-C-C-C-C (count them -- 18 C's or 18 carbons)

    The active tissues (muscles and organs) use these free fatty acids as a source of fuel. To do so, however, the 18-carbon chain must first break down into nine 2-carbon fragments. The 2-carbon compounds are called acetyl-CoA, the chemical used by the body to produce energy.

    In starvation, or in a low-carbohydrate diet, insulin levels decrease. The ***primary*** purpose of insulin is to stop the release of stored fat from the fat cell, limiting the breakdown of the free fatty acid storage form, triglyceride. Insulin's ***secondary*** purpose is to clear sugar from the blood. Remember this order, most doctors think these jobs are reversed.

The Complete Scoop on the Low-Carbohydrate Diet

Glucagon is the other pancreatic hormone that controls fuel flow and its actions oppose those of insulin; it increases the liver's ketone-making machinery while insulin controls the delivery of fat from the fat cells to the liver.

Carbohydrate intake **increases** insulin release and **decreases** glucagon release from the pancreas. Starvation and low-carbohydrate diets **decrease** the release of insulin and **increase** the rate of glucagon release. In the absence of insulin, the fat cell increases its rate of triglyceride breakdown. In response to this breakdown, free fatty acids leave the fat cell and enter the blood.

It is, however, the **ratio** between glucagon and insulin that determines the direction of fuel flow, into storage or burning. The type of food eaten controls this ratio, with carbohydrate eating driving fuels into storage and away from burning (food is not the only control -- exercise affects these hormones too).

The blood doesn't like high amounts of free fatty acids. So, the liver sucks them up and burns them. The enzymes in the liver slash the 18-carbon chain into nine 2-carbon fragments. The liver, then, recombines two 2-carbon fragments into a chain that's now four carbons long. This is a ketone body, and the liver then releases it into the blood. Free fatty acids are more toxic to the body than ketones and the body, therefore, more readily tolerates higher levels of ketones than free fatty acids.

Ketones in the blood enter the active tissues, where they're split again, into the two 2-carbon acetyl-CoA fragments. Acetyl-CoA provides the source of energy for all cells.

Many claim that ketones are waste products of fat metabolism, products arising from partially burned fat.

This is absolutely untrue. Ketones are important products in the body's metabolism of fuels.

In several experiments, researchers exposed muscle cells to ketones, free fatty acids, or glucose (blood sugar) to test the cell's preferences for the different fuels. The result was that muscle cells chose to burn ketones as their primary fuel! After 12 days of starvation, or low-carbohydrate dieting, ketones represent 75% of the fuel used by the brain and nervous system, which cannot burn free fatty acids. Fat, therefore, is delivered to these active tissues as ketones.

Fat is the Preferred Fuel of the Body -- Not Carbohydrate

Throughout the day, in normal activities and in light to moderate exercise, the body uses fuel to meet its energy needs and both fat and carbohydrates can supply this fuel. In high-carbohydrate diets, the brain and the nervous system burn glucose. They can't burn free fatty acids. In a high-carbohydrate diet, almost no ketones form because the source of the ketones is free fatty acids (released from the fat tissue). In the high-carbohydrate diet then, the supply of free fatty acids is reduced because insulin inhibits their release from the fat cell (not entirely because the longer time away from the last meal leads to a decreasing release of insulin which removes the brakes stopping the fat cell's release of free fatty acids). In contrast, during a low-carbohydrate diet, the brain switches to burning ketones.

The current "folk wisdom" of the man in the street -- and among athletes and scientists as well -- is that carbohydrates are the body's preferred source of fuel.

Not true. The body **prefers** to burn fat. One can force his body to burn more carbohydrate by eating more carbohydrate, but this also forces the body to produce more fat from carbohydrate. Remember, though, the body prefers to burn fat. Given the chance, it will burn fat all day long.

In a resting body, fat provides most of the energy, regardless of diet type. This is because muscles and organs prefer to burn fat. As the carbohydrate content in the diet decreases, the brain and nervous system burn more fat in the form of ketones. For all people, **up to 80-90% of total energy at rest, and 50-75% during exercise, comes from fat, not carbohydrate.**

How the Body "Burns" Food

The body processes food by moving it through enzymes and enzyme pathways. Like a bucket brigade of fire fighters, the process shuttles food along in a series of steps. Each step transforms the food into a different chemical. During the shuttling process, the body extracts the potential energy. The food moves along these pathways and releases its energy until it's sucked dry.

The body's cells have different enzyme pathways for burning fats and carbohydrates. Ultimately, after breaking-down to a common biochemical, it then enters a common pathway for its final use. But to get to this point, fats and carbohydrates follow their own specific paths of breakdown.

The pathway that burns fats **controls** the pathway that burns carbohydrates. ***It's not the other way round; carbohydrate burning doesn't regulate fat burning***. If cells burn fat, a signal from fat burning slows carbohydrate use. These signals slow-down the enzymes that control the rate of carbohydrate burning. The result is that carbohydrate burning slows.

Body Composition Changes: Low-Carbohydrate vs. Low-Fat

We've seen how low- and high-carbohydrate diets affect the body at the cellular level. Are these cellular changes a reflection of what happens at the whole body level? They should be. Let's find out.

Dr. Betty Alford tested sedentary and overweight adult women for 3 weeks. She fed three different groups either a 25%-, 45%-, or 75%-carbohydrate diet. The total calorie intake for each woman was held constant at 1,200 calories a day. Dr. Alford published the results of her study in 1990 in the *Journal of the American Dietetic Association*.

She stated that all diets contributed favorably to improved health. There weren't any differences in cholesterol and triglycerides in any groups. She evaluated whether changes from the three varied carbohydrate diets were statistically different. They weren't. She looked to see if bodyweight, fat mass, and Lean Body Mass changed. (In the chart, CHO is an acronym for carbohydrate.)

	25% CHO	45% CHO	75% CHO
Bodyweight loss (lbs.)	14.1	12.3	10.8
Body Fat loss (lbs.)	12.0	10.7	7.9
Lean Mass loss (lbs.)	2.1	1.6	2.6
% Lean Mass loss	17%	15%	33%

I've provided the table, above, to help us observe what I call the "practical significance" of these results. We see that 4.1 pounds more fat was lost on the 25%-carbohydrate diet than on the 75%-carbohydrate diet.

Even the 45%-carbohydrate dieters fared quite well. Note the similarity between the two low-carbohydrate diets. The 25%-carbohydrate diet is at the threshold of being a true low-carbohydrate diet. Therefore, responses to 25%-carbohydrate are not dramatically different than the responses to a 45%-carbohydrate diet. The major influence in this study was the reduction of calories to 1,200 a day. This large reduction in calories overrides many of the effects by changes in carbohydrate composition.

Dr. Gerald Reaven published a study of adult men who were fed a 1,000 calorie, 15%-carbohydrate diet, or a 1,000 calorie, 45%-carbohydrate diet.

	15% CHO (53% fat)	**45% CHO (26% fat)**
Weight Loss (lbs.)	17.6	15.4
Fat Loss	19.8	15.4
Lean Body Mass	+ 2.2	0.0

The subjects performed one hour of aerobic exercise and one hour of underwater physical activity a day for six weeks. The changes in the subjects were not statistically significant. My less "scientific" standard of "practical significance" supports the value of a 15%-carbohydrate diet.

Why? It works best because the 15%-carbohydrate diet promoted fat loss and increased muscle mass (Lean Body Mass, although I assume it was muscle because organs don't change much in response to exercise). This was only a six-week study. From a practical viewpoint, if it had lasted six months, or one year, the results would have been more impressive. Unfortunately, there are no long-term studies to support my conclusion. I'm relying on my own many years of experience working with the low-carbohydrate diet for my source of information and experience.

Dr. Reaven's study used 1,000 calories and a 15%-carbohydrate diet compared with Dr. Alford's use of 1,200 calories and 25%- and 45%- low-carbohydrate diet. Decreasing carbohydrate by another 10% (and 30%) of total calories led to more fat loss and stimulated an increase in Lean Body Mass in the study by Dr. Reaven, with exercise likely contributing to the increases in Lean Body Mass.

Adding several pounds of muscle and losing several pounds of fat make a huge difference in one's physical appearance. We've seen that low-carbohydrate eating decreases fat manufacturing at the **cellular level**. We've also seen, now, that low-carbohydrate eating decreases fat at the **whole body level**. These two profound changes demonstrate the value of the low-carbohydrate diet: it promotes fat loss and muscle gain. Later in this chapter, I'll describe the biochemistry underlying this response.

In another study of a low-carbohydrate diet, the outcome variable included changes in body composition. Dr. Charlotte Young of Cornell University tested low-carbohydrate diets, varying the amounts of carbohydrate. Here are the results for weight loss, fat loss, and lean loss.

	23% CHO	13% CHO	7% CHO
Weight loss (lbs.)	24.6	27.1	34.3
Fat loss (lbs.)	18.5	22.4	32.8
Lean loss (lbs.)	6.1	4.7	1.5
% Wt. loss as Fat	75%	83%	95%
% Wt. loss as Lean	25%	17%	5%

This was a 1,800 calorie a day diet. It lasted 9 weeks. As the carbohydrate content of the diet dropped, the percent of the bodyweight lost as fat increased.

The pattern of tissue loss in the 23%-carbohydrate diet was similar to that indicated in the graph located in the body composition chapter. That graph showed that bodyweight losses are composed of both Fat Mass and Lean Body Mass. These two tissues are companions when one losses bodyweight: the ***typical*** pattern of tissue loss is 25% loss as Lean Body Mass and a 75% loss as Fat Mass.

But, look how the 7%-carbohydrate diet, in the chart, above, up-staged that normal relationship between losses of Fat Mass and Lean Body Mass. The low-carbohydrate diet is powerful enough to overcome the body's normal body composition response to bodyweight loss. I discovered this powerful effect when I switched to the low-carbohydrate diet myself. This diet gave me the control I was looking for in gaining muscle and losing fat!

Why Do Low-Carbohydrate Dieters Lose More Bodyweight than High-Carbohydrate Dieters?

Dr. U. Rabast confirmed that the low-carbohydrate diet increases ***bodyweight*** loss. He studied 21 obese adults using 3 different diets: all three diets were low in calories and two were low-carbohydrate diets and the third diet was a high-carbohydrate (67%-carbohydrate and 12%-fat). Weight loss was 21 pounds on the high-carbohydrate diet, 25.1 pounds on one low-carbohydrate diet, and 27.5 pounds on the other low-carbohydrate diet.

All low-carbohydrate studies have the same result: the low-carbohydrate group loses more bodyweight than those eating a high-carbohydrate diet. Researchers, however, often credit this increased loss in ***bodyweight*** to a specific loss in ***fat*** tissue. One cannot infer, however, solely from changes in bodyweight that the body lost more fat. The major problem, then, in these early studies is that researchers did exactly that; they inferred that bodyweight losses solely reflected changes in fat and lean. But, there's another explanation for more bodyweight loss in low-carbohydrate dieting: water loss.

In the mid-1950's Drs. Kekwick and Pawan were the first to observe higher bodyweight losses with a carbohydrate-restricted diet compared with a high-carbohydrate diet. These two medical doctors proposed the idea of "special metabolic factors" instead of the simpler explanation of increases in water loss for the higher bodyweight losses, particularly in the first two weeks of following a low-carbohydrate diet. Their work set off a firestorm of criticism leading to much scientific research during the next quarter-century in an attempt to resolve whether the increased bodyweight loss was accounted for by water or by fat. It turned out that it was mostly water and some fat. Let's see how the story unfolded.

Changes in **bodyweight** are <u>unreliable</u> for analyzing the changes in body composition: muscle, fat, and water, during a weight reduction program. And, with the use of two-compartment body composition testing, instead of three-compartment that measures water along with Lean Body Mass and Fat Mass, errors occur. Variations in water content during weight loss are a difficult barrier to understanding changes in muscle and fat, particularly in the first seven to twenty days of a diet. The failure to understand this concept was the major limitation to those early scientific studies. This also tripped up Atkins.

One of the inevitable after-effects of ending a low calorie, low-carbohydrate diet is rapid weight regain. Rapid weight regain is not a common characteristic of ending a low calorie, high-carbohydrate diet. Researchers finally figured out that the rapid weight regain after ending the low-carbohydrate diet reset the body water levels that had been reduced solely from carbohydrate restriction. Many researchers have argued that this observation is proof that carbohydrate restriction leads to more water loss than that occurring by following a low calorie, high-carbohydrate diet.

The studies of Kekwick and Pawan lasted only a few days. During studies of several days, changes in water loss (or gain) account for most of the variations in bodyweight. Carbohydrate-restriction leads to more water loss in short studies than a high-carbohydrate diet. Once researchers extended the diet trials, bodyweight loss was often, but not always, equal among the high-carbohydrate and low-carbohydrate groups. This was more proof that the high, rapid, early bodyweight loss in low-carbohydrate dieters was water and not fat.

As the decades passed, researchers used more sophisticated studies of body composition to measure changes during bodyweight loss. These studies confirmed that water losses arising from using the low-carbohydrate diet accounted for most of the increased bodyweight losses in the early stages. Low-carbohydrate shills use this, however, to mislead their followers who believe that weight loss reflected by changes in the bathroom scale reflect losses of fat tissue. Boy, are they mistaken. And so are the fraudulent hucksters that profit from conning the purchasers of their so-called miracle program.

Studies do confirm, importantly, that the low-carbohydrate diet does lead to more fat loss and less muscle loss than a high-carbohydrate diet over longer time periods. This fat loss, however, does not account for the total amount of bodyweight that was lost. Far from it as a greater proportion of the early weight loss is water weight. And some of this bodyweight loss remains over longer times because one eating a low-carbohydrate diet carries less water in his body. So, even in studies of long duration, such as Dr. Young's above, the greater loss in bodyweight and supposedly in fat may be actually be water losses. Without directly measuring water, it's impossible to tell.

Following a low-carbohydrate diet leads to significant losses of water, some increased loss of fat, and preservation of muscle. Initially, water losses represent the largest part of the bodyweight loss. The high-carbohydrate diet does not cause the same level of water loss or fat loss as does the low-carbohydrate diet. It's difficult to distinguish the percent of the body mass that is lost as water or as fat because the body composition methods aren't sophisticated enough to do so. That's one of the reasons why it was so difficult to settle the controversy.

The studies with animals, however, provide strong evidence that low-carbohydrate eating causes increased fat loss. To analyze the animals' body composition, researchers kill the animals and chemically analyze their carcasses. This technique provides an exact measure of the fat, lean, and water content of the animal's body. There's little error with the use of this technique.

I've already cited several convincing animal studies proving that the low-carbohydrate diet leads to more losses of fat than the high-carbohydrate diet; here's another good one. Rats were fed two diets that differed in carbohydrate content. One group ate 0%-carbohydrates; and the other group ate 66%-carbohydrate. The carcass fat content of the 0%-carbohydrate group was 13% less than that in the 66%-carbohydrate group.

The important point in the above pages is that most of the higher **bodyweight** loss from the use of a low-carbohydrate diet during the early weeks of dieting occurs because of increased water loss. For **body composition**, however, there's more fat loss and muscle preservation by using the low-carbohydrate diet. The low-carbohydrate diet will outperform the high-carbohydrate diet in respect to fat loss.

It's important, however, to realize that most of the rapid, early bodyweight losses are water. One must not be fooled that this bodyweight loss is fat. And even with the increased fat losses, these changes won't reflect a loss of 100 pounds of fat on a low-carbohydrate diet and none on a low-fat diet. After several months and a loss of considerable bodyweight the low-carbohydrate diet may help the dieter lose about 5-10 more pounds of fat than if he followed a low-fat diet. Good? Yes. This is my technique of putting-the-numbers-to-it to get a real handle in what is actually happening. The way most people talk, they act like the fat is just going to melt off the body and completely disappear. No, sorry, that's not the way it works. And if the low-carbohydrate dieter doesn't pay attention to the calories he consumes, he'll lose nothing and often, even, gain weight. You gotta' pay attention, first, to the Energy Balance Equation.

Insulin Increases Eating and Fat Storage

The hormonal stimulus causing the reduced carcass fat in the low-carbohydrate fed animals is the low levels of glucose and insulin and the high level of glucagon. These two hormones control the use of fat and carbohydrate. High insulin leads to fat storage; low insulin leads to fat release and glucagon kicks-up the ketone producing machinery in the liver.

High insulin levels are a characteristic feature of obesity. Administration of insulin to experimental animals, eating what they wanted, caused a large increase in food intake and, hence, obesity. Insulin, acting directly on the feeding center in the brain and indirectly by clearing the blood of fuel, stimulated **appetite** and **eating**. Remember, it's all about calories.

Researchers wondered whether insulin caused an increase in fat mass, independent of eating behavior. Here was the question: If calorie intake was the same, would insulin, by itself, make the animal fat?

Their results demonstrated that increases in body fat occurred as muscle and water decreased. Insulin caused animals to gain fat and lose muscle. All groups had been fed **exactly** the same number of calories through feed tubes inserted into their stomachs, a method that removed the effect of variations in calorie intake on any changes in body composition. **Bodyweight** gains were similar among the groups.

Amazingly, insulin treatment of animals that ate the same number of calories as animals not treated with insulin led to increased body fat and decreased muscle. **The Energy Balance Equation was still obeyed as fuels came from different sources.** If fuel is stored in body fat, energy must come from somewhere, if we control calorie intake, to meet energy requirements. The Energy Balance Equation must be satisfied. Here, the muscles provided the fuel as insulin drove calories into fat storage away from burning in the active tissues.

Low-carbohydrate eating reduces insulin release, and high-carbohydrate eating increases insulin release. The body composition changes occurring from eating a low-carbohydrate diet include the preservation of muscle and loss of fat. Conversely, a high-carbohydrate diet increases insulin release, fat gain, and muscle loss. This body composition effect even occurs whether consuming the number of calories needed or consuming fewer, although its degree varies with calorie intake. A lower calorie intake will lead to smaller changes. These fluctuations are a function of energy-partitioning. I'll discuss in detail the role that energy-partitioning has in body composition, hunger, and appetite later.

How Low Do Carbohydrate Grams Have to Go?

It's astounding that one can gain fat while losing bodyweight, but this is a direct effect of carbohydrates.

To reverse these effects so that fat loss occurs and muscle increases, one must eat a low-carbohydrate diet. These positive effects from a low-carbohydrate diet begin when carbohydrate intake drops to less than approximately 25% of total calories. Since there's no research on this, I've had to estimate this percentage from my extensive studies and experience.

Consistently, I observed that fat storage occurred when carbohydrate content was 25-30% or higher of total calories. Below this amount, fat storage from carbohydrate slowed, and fat burning increased. Obviously, an individual's calorie intake affects these variations in the storage of fat from carbohydrate. Although I'll give the details of my version of the low-carbohydrate diet in a later chapter, you can see that you have a much wider range for carbohydrate gram ingestion for this diet type to be effective than that offered by the misinformed "experts" (such as Atkins) who promote a very restrictive, low, and virtually impossible-to-maintain daily carbohydrate intake.

Is a 0%-carbohydrate diet the best? I don't know. We need further studies to find out the best percentage. Studies of Alaskan sled racing dogs have found that decreasing the percentage of carbohydrate in the dogs' diet improved their performance. The best performance was on a 0%-carbohydrate diet. Here's the problem: few people ever maintain an extremely low or 0%-carbohydrate diet. It's just too hard to do. I maintained a 0%-carbohydrate diet for four months, but that was it.

I argue that the **combination** of carbohydrates and fat, our typical diet, is the most fattening. Insulin, the fat storage hormone, increases from eating carbohydrates.

The result of high blood insulin and glucose levels is a stimulation of storage of both carbohydrates and fat as body fat. When carbohydrate (hence insulin) is low, fat from the diet burns as energy. As long as carbohydrate intake is low, fat comes out of the fat cells and circulates in the blood, available for burning as fuel by muscle and organs.

Over the last 40 years, I've tried every diet imaginable, including the vegetarian life-style for 3 years. I followed a high complex carbohydrate diet for many years, and a high-protein/high-carbohydrate diet. I've done a low-carbohydrate diet with high-protein; that's what I use now. Low-carbohydrate is the winner. When I finally lowered the carbohydrate and **calories** enough, I lost about 6 pounds of fat and increased muscle by about 6 pounds.

My advocacy of this diet doesn't imply that I think it's more important than the Energy Balance Equation. It's not: the best results in the control of weight come from balancing what one eats and burns.

This is very little compared with changes that accompany an exercise program or decreases in total calorie intake. *I see the low-carbohydrate diet as fine-tuning.* These changes in body composition are, undoubtedly, more important to athletes. In athletes, a percent or two increase in performance is enough to determine who wins or loses.

We still need much more research to define the optimal percent of carbohydrates in the diet and the length of time to adapt to burning fat. Unfortunately, most scientists working with low-carbohydrate diets never drop the carbohydrates low enough. They don't get to the point where the body switches over to maximal fat burning. I feel that carbohydrate intake must be below

25% of total calories before the positive effects begin. Rarely do researchers drop below 35%, and an intake of a 30%-carbohydrate is too high to push the body into a maximal fat burning zone. The Zone program by Dr. Barry Sears is 40%-carbohydrate; that's much too high to drive fat burning.

Regardless of what one chooses to do about diet composition, the most important consideration is the Energy Balance Equation. However, one must understand this: to get optimal results, one must follow a low-carbohydrate diet.

How the Low-Carbohydrate Diet Works Metabolically

This diet works because it obeys the body's laws of fuel metabolism and hormonal control. The mechanism of the low-carbohydrate diet is not a guess, not an opinion; it's based on biochemical facts. The low-fat diet fails because its framework doesn't rely on biochemical facts. The low-fat diet defies what we scientists know about cellular biochemistry.

The body releases insulin to control its level of blood glucose (blood sugar). Insulin's primary function, as I've said, is to control the release of fat from the fat cell. Its secondary job is to maintain the blood glucose level within very narrow limits, which insulin does by storing some (a little) glucose as glycogen (a chain of glucose molecules) and most of it as fat. Glycogen storage amounts are small. The liver can hold ¼ pound and the muscles hold ¾ pound of glycogen. The body contains 60 times more fat than carbohydrate reserves.

Glucose not used immediately (for energy and for storage in the liver and muscles as glycogen) converts into fat. This conversion occurs both in the liver and in adipose tissue, but mostly in adipose tissue.

The most important action of insulin, however, is to slow the release of fat from fat cells. It's also the most powerful hormone stimulating the conversion of carbohydrate to fat. I say this again and again because I want this fact burned into your memory.

Remember: insulin is a fat-making hormone. High insulin levels from eating a high-carbohydrate diet, along with lots of calories, makes you fat. High insulin also stimulates hunger and you eat too much. It's that easy.

And if you eat fat along with your carbohydrates, the fat stores as fat too. No, it doesn't go directly to body fat. That's the simple, super-market magazine tale. Ingested fat is first broken down and then built back up into a different fat (chylomicrons) which are burned or stored. Fat making enzymes do this. The continued eating of a high-carbohydrate diet locks the fat inside the fat cell.

When insulin is low (as in the low-carbohydrate diet), fat cells release fat. Organs and muscles burn fat for energy. **One eats less**, loses weight, and feels great. When insulin is high (as in the high-carbohydrate diet), LPL is low in muscle and high in fat cells. The fat load in the blood is then forced into storage. The fat cells suck up the carbohydrate, converting it to fat. Conversely, when insulin is low (as in the low-carbohydrate diet), LPL is high in muscle and low in fat. Now fat from the blood goes into muscle where it's burned for energy. This satisfies the muscles' and organs' need for food and reduces food intake. That's because the muscles are no longer starving.

Restricted eating and dieting increases the fat making capacity of the body upon re-feeding carbohydrates. These changes account for the enormous failure rates experienced by dieters attempting to maintain their reduced-weight. But, you now know how to overcome this problem. The cat is out of the bag, and everyone can take advantage of the **Biological control of weight loss and weight control**. Forget about the Willpower fight. The **Power of Nature** is now in your hands.

This is a very important chapter for gaining a thorough understanding about how diet composition impacts upon appetite, hunger, bodyweight, and body composition. This is Chapter 13 in the 600-page UDS book and that Chapter is available for download at my site if you want to look very deeply into this topic and all of the regulatory mechanisms involved. I simply could not keep that total content from Chapter 13 in UDS Lite if I wanted it to be Lite. You are seeing, of course, why UDS is such a long book. It had to be to provide the most detailed analysis of bodyweight regulation ever written.

Chapter 10

Dietary Control of Appetite and Hunger

I want to summarize, here, what you've learned in the last several chapters so as to eliminate any confusion about what type of foods control appetite and hunger. On the Energy-In side of the Equation, it's **appetite** and **hunger** that affect bodyweight. If one wants to control bodyweight, then one must control his food intake. The important point is this: for the Energy-In side of the Energy Balance Equation, the most powerful things to control, then, are **appetite** and **hunger**. The most effective way to do this is with **Biological** methods, not with displays of heroic **Willpower** and Self-control.

Most people, even most scientists, believe that the high-fat content of modern diets is the primary cause of obesity. I challenge that view. Many scientific studies have evaluated the effects of low-fat foods on weight control, and the results of these studies have proved to be sorely disappointing.

Energy-Partitioning and Food Intake

There's no doubt that diet composition affects food intake (by increasing, or decreasing, appetite and hunger). But how?

The effect of diet composition on food intake depends upon whether the body **stores** food in the adipose tissue or **burns** food in the active tissues. Studies show that food burned for energy satisfies appetite and reduces food intake. If, instead, food is stored in fat tissue, it doesn't satisfy appetite and, as a consequence, food intake increases to meet the calorie needs of the active tissues.

Dietary Control of Appetite and Hunger

Energy-partitioning is important because it dictates the availability of fuel to produce energy. Scientists believe that energy-partitioning of carbohydrate and fat is a primary factor in the control of food intake. The hypothesis that energy-partitioning controls food intake is termed the **Metabolic Control of Food Intake**. The Energy-In side (what we eat) of the Energy Balance Equation is affected by energy-partitioning.

The body's regulatory systems are geared to provide calories to meet the active tissues' needs. Any disruption in the supply of calories to the active tissues cripples their ability to function. Energy-partitioning, through the storage of calories into fat tissue, interrupts the delivery of fuel to the active tissues: the muscles and organs. Regulatory systems must counteract reductions in fuel delivery to the active tissues by increasing supplies. To do so, the regulatory systems drive appetite and hunger and push the body to increase its food intake.

Fat and carbohydrate disposal into storage as body fat, on the one hand, or into muscles and organs for burning, on the other, sends different signals to the brain. Therefore, the site of fuel disposal influences eating behavior and the type of signal received by the brain increases or decreases food intake.

Enzymes control the flow of fuels either into adipose tissue or into muscles and organs. **The type of food consumed dictates the way the enzymes distribute food energy** and dictates hormonal changes, which also exert control over enzymes in that there are specific enzymes and metabolic pathways for handling fats and carbohydrates. The sum of these changes dictates energy-partitioning.

Carbohydrates increase the enzymes and metabolic pathways leading to fat making from carbohydrate. Fuel storage into fat tissue increases the eating response and fuel burning in muscle and organs decreases the eating response. These shifts in energy-partitioning, therefore, impact the Energy Balance Equation because food that is stored isn't available for burning!

It's clear, at this juncture, that energy-partitioning is one of the most powerful controls of food intake. Obesity partly arises because of the energy-partitioning of carbohydrate foods into fat storage, which increases appetite, hunger, and eating. I believe that all the biochemical research over the last 140 years provides the basis for my conclusion.

This explanation moves away from a focus on the calories that <u>enter</u> <u>the</u> <u>mouth</u> and toward the <u>metabolism</u> and <u>disposal</u> of the metabolic fuels in the active tissues as the primary mechanism that controls food intake.

Calories from all sources are available for energy production, including those that enter the mouth and those that are already a part of the body's tissues. Body fuels that serve as a source of calories include body fat and muscles and organs.

In the Metabolic Control of Food Intake, control of calorie intake isn't related to the calories one eats, but depends on whether calories are available for burning. Let's discuss this idea in detail.

It's calories BURNED <u>as</u> <u>energy</u>, not <u>calories</u> <u>EATEN</u>, that determines appetite, hunger, and how much one eats. The calories that enter the mouth and stomach don't control food intake. *How the body disposes of the calories it eats, either into fat for storage or into muscles and organs for burning, determines food intake.*

These discoveries show that the control of food intake is a complex process. Food intake control relies on the integration of signals from many feedback loops. **But, ultimately, the primary factor controlling food intake is the <u>relationship</u> between the <u>storage</u> and <u>burning</u> of calories.** All evidence suggests that an integrated signal arising from the storage or burning of **both** glucose and fatty acids controls food intake. And it is the availability of fuel for the active tissues that provides the strongest signal for controlling food intake (unless body tissues become depleted; that's a stronger signal).

For the body to *draw* from the energy contained in food, these fuels must be metabolized and burned. The entry of calories into the mouth and their circulation in the blood isn't enough. In the process of breaking down food, there's a give-and-take relation between the use of fats and glucose which means that changes in the burning of one are counteracted by changes in the burning of the other. This interrelationship between the body's use of these two fuels is the key feature of the Metabolic Control of Food Intake.

The Relationship Between Fat and Carbohydrate Metabolism Determines Food Intake

As described earlier, eating carbohydrates causes the body to convert some portion of the carbohydrates into storage as fat, a well known response of the body to eating carbohydrates. Fuel stored, instead of being burned, starves the active tissues which then signal the brain to drive eating.

> **The starving tissues want food! They don't care that you have already eaten and think yourself to be well fed. Instead, the food you ate went to fat storage, but the muscles and organs remain hungry.**

We've learned that feeding a high-fat diet to animals and to people produces overeating and obesity, **but only when** this "so-called" high-fat diet is also high in carbohydrate.

Scientific researchers rarely state or even understand this fact. A diet that is high-fat **and** low-carbohydrate doesn't produce overeating: To produce overeating, the diet must be **both** high-fat **and** high-carbohydrate. It's eating a **combination** high-fat, high-carbohydrate diet that drives hyperphagia (ravenous overeating) and obesity.

So, eating a typical high-fat diet -- the so-called mixed diet that's also high in carbohydrates -- directs both glucose and fat into storage. This diet directs fuel away from burning in the active tissues, and provides less hunger satisfaction. Unfortunately, the conversion of fuel into fat turns-on the hunger drive. You then eat too much, more than you need, and get fatter yet.

The defining characteristic of consuming a mixed diet is that one becomes obese in the face of starvation because carbohydrate eating shoves fuels into storage in the fat tissue turning it away from use by the active tissues. The active tissues, now starving, send out powerful feeding signals to the brain. These signals drive the hunger response. This is a no-win situation because Biology always overcomes Willpower.

In a person who has lost weight, fat burning occurs at a slower rate than it did before weight reduction. Fat burning is also less when comparing a person who has lost weight to people who have never been overweight. Scientists have blamed the slow rate of fat burning for the tendency of persons who have lost weight to regain weight after dieting.

Dietary Control of Appetite and Hunger

The experiments leading to the observation of slower fat burning in weight reduced persons always tested this response while feeding <u>mixed</u> diets that are both high in carbohydrate and fat. It's my contention that this observation is strictly related to the effects of the mixed diet.

People who have lost weight are **highly primed** to convert carbohydrate-to-fat because the body wants to return to its higher bodyweight. All of the weight reduced person's enzymes want to store food as fat. The after-effect of the bodyweight loss is an acceleration of energy-partitioning of fuel into body fat and a mixed diet rapidly causes fat **storage** and less fat **burning**. The reason the researchers observed less fat burning in persons who have lost weight is because weight reduced people are geared to store their calories as fat; that's what the body wants to do in its effort to replenish its Fat Mass.

So, of course, the person who has lost weight burns less fat than before losing weight because his metabolic machinery to store carbohydrate and fat as fat has been turned on. He's all revved up to store everything because of restricted feeding and bodyweight loss.

Consuming a low-fat/high-carbohydrate diet, or a mixed diet, is an absolute **DEATHBLOW** to a person who has lost weight. His fat tissue is ready to suck up circulating fuels, desiring to restore itself to its previous high fat level. All the metabolic machinery, including the drive to eat and the enzymatic pathways, ramp up to produce fat from any fuel. Overcoming these drives by Willpower is virtually impossible.

Post-starvation obesity after food restriction is an **expected** response. Hyperphagia (ravenous overeating) is a biological drive to return the organism to its bodyweight Set-Point. Overeating is turned-off only when the body's Fat Mass and Lean Body Mass have returned to pre-weight loss levels unless we **shut this process down** with special techniques. Most people don't use these techniques and this is why 95-98% of people fail to maintain their weight loss.

This shift in energy-partitioning toward storage is independent of changes in food intake! **Increases in fat storage occur before one begins overeating.** This is a very important fact. It demonstrates that energy-partitioning of fuels into fat storage happens **before** one overeats and the storage of fuels away from burning is the **reason** and **drive** for overeating. This response has been observed in every animal model studied, including more than 143 different studies. **Fat storage, therefore, precedes overeating.**

So overeating and obesity both result from a failure of fuels to burn in the active tissues. The signals driving overeating arise from the starving active tissue mass. In this model, there is no lack of food from the outside. Unfortunately, the food one has eaten is gobbled up by and locked away in the adipose tissue. It's now unavailable to the active tissues, and in a real sense, **the individual becomes obese in the face of starvation.**

Chapter 11

Crushing the Criticism Against the Low-Carbohydrate Diet

Challenges to the Low-Carbohydrate Diet

Many scientists criticize the low-carbohydrate diet plan as contrary to everything that medicine and nutritional science hold dear. Their virulent attack derives from many misbeliefs they hold about the low-carbohydrate diet including the following:

1) The diet is unbalanced, both in energy composition and in vitamins and minerals.
2) It puts the body into a dangerous state of ketosis, possibly leading to death.
3) It increases the risk of heart disease by increasing saturated fats, blood triglycerides, and cholesterol.
4) It leads to fatigue.
5) It can raise uric acid levels, deplete calcium from bones, cause acidosis, and cause kidney problems.

First, they're right about one point -- the nutritional balance. The diet is not based on the accepted standards for protein, fat, and carbohydrate. So what? Just because our nutrition institutions and dietary experts claim that they "know" the ideal diet doesn't make that claim true. For example, in complete contradiction to the politically correct diet recommendations made today, many years ago the Arctic explorer Vilhjalmur Stefansson lived on an exclusive meat diet, off and on, for 10 years. He had no negative health effects, only positive ones. During 1928-1929, he and another explorer underwent rigorous medical evaluations for one year while eating an exclusive meat diet.

Crushing the Criticism Against the Low-Carbohydrate Diet

Many scientists expected them to drop dead within 3 weeks, but they didn't. Stefansson and his fellow explorer remained in perfect health. In fact, they became healthier. The attending doctor, a well-regarded specialist, said that the most remarkable outcome was the fact that nothing remarkable had materialized. I know this is shocking, but these are the facts. The results of these dietary experiments and medical evaluations were published in the *Journal of Biological Chemistry* for anyone who wants to corroborate them.

Recommendations are just that -- recommendations. They can be wrong. There's a large database supporting the value of low-carbohydrate dieting, but most critics of low-carbohydrate diets simply ignore it (or, because of a lack of effort, fail to even become aware of it). The low-carbohydrate diet, high in meat and high in fat, has been around a lot longer than the 30-year-old "politically correct" low-fat diet.

More than forty years ago, Dr. John Yudkin addressed many of the criticisms against the low-carbohydrate diet. He evaluated the effect of low-carbohydrate eating on nutrient intake, comparing the low-carbohydrate diet to a nutrient-balanced low calorie diet. The key advantage that Yudkin attributed to low-carbohydrate eating was the ease with which people cut back on total calorie intake because they weren't hungry.

In his study of low-carbohydrate diets, he calculated that the vitamin and mineral intake was adequate. ***In fact, it was actually better on a low-carbohydrate diet than on the so-called "balanced diet" that had the same number of calories***. He also found that the diet wasn't harmful to one's health and that it met all of one's nutritional needs.

The total fat intake in a low-carbohydrate diet is within the "Establishment's" normal, recommended

healthy ranges for saturated fat too. A low-carbohydrate diet isn't high in saturated fat, despite the critics' outcry. This, most likely, results from the fact that people consume less food. The critics who claim that the diet is nutritionally unbalanced are wrong. Dr. Yudkin used this diet for over 35 years with no subjects reporting hunger or any other ill effects.

Contrary to what many believe, there are many scientific publications about low-carbohydrate dieting. I have spent years gathering the published works in this area, and all the papers come to the same conclusion:

1) The diet is adequate in all nutrients except calories.
2) It's simple to follow, at and away from home.
3) If you choose, you can use it as your normal life-long eating pattern for weight maintenance and health.
4) It doesn't increase blood lipids (fats) or the risk of heart disease.
5) And most important, it reduces hunger and fatigue.

The First Major Attacks

The first major attack of the low-carbohydrate diet occurred after the 1972 publication of Dr. Atkins <u>Diet Revolution</u>. Published in the *Journal of the American Medical Association*, the Council on Foods and Nutrition critiqued Atkins' low-carbohydrate regimen.

In this section, I review many of the criticisms posited against the low-carbohydrate diet over the years, responding to each one (big UDS covers them all and Chapter 15 is a downloadable e-chapter). The major attacks against the low-carbohydrate diet have continued unabated since the early 1970's. Since several writers have proposed low-carbohydrate diets in the last decade, attacks of it have increased.

Therefore, the time has come for someone to set the record straight and that's exactly what I'm about to do. No one else has shouldered the task of correcting the myths surrounding the low-carbohydrate diet. Critics of the diet continue ranting the same incorrect and misinformed allegations they've shouted for almost 30 years. One would think that one scientist, somewhere, who's critical of the low-carbohydrate diet, would check whether or not the criticisms are really true. But they don't. Instead, these scientists endlessly circulate the same false claims, like a computer virus, infecting people's minds with false information. They never attempt to validate whether their low-carbohydrate damning claims are, in fact, true!

The Critics' Claims

Critics point out that modern versions of the low-carbohydrate are neither new nor innovative. This is true. Most low-carbohydrate plans have common features: 1) a low to very low-carbohydrate content, 2) no restriction of protein and fat, and 3) unrestricted calorie intake.

The third feature, unrestricted calorie intake, is a common feature served-up by low-carbohydrate supporters and writers. Pennington, 1953, published *Treatment of Obesity with Calorically Unrestricted Diets*. The Air Force diet, 1960, also promoted unrestricted calories. Taller, 1961, wrote Calories Don't Count. The Drinking Man's Diet appeared in 1964 followed in 1967 by the Stillman diet, with both books promoting the idea that calories aren't important in weight control. Dr. Atkins' 1972 release, Dr. Atkins Diet Revolution, has been the most successful in sales volume of the books listed, above, and he has been the most devoted supporter of the idea that calories don't count.

All of these books and programs were remarkable in their agreement with, and emphasis of, the notion that calories don't count. Even Atkins' 1999 release continues to emphasize that calories don't count. The actress, Suzanne Somers, also makes a similar claim in her recent book.

Criticism: Calories Don't Count

Therefore, the main outcry by the scientific experts against the low-carbohydrate diet is against its authors' claim that calories don't count. This criticism is, in fact, right-on the mark. These authors who claim that calories don't count are all wrong, dead wrong; calories do count.

This **critical mistake** by the low-carbohydrate authors has provided their critics with a powerful weapon. The critics figured that, if these writers so profoundly misunderstood the most accepted and least arguable dictum in nutritional science, that they were wrong about everything else they said about the diet too. The low-carbohydrate authors, as a result of denying the Energy Balance Equation, **tarnished their credibility** on any issue related to nutrition.

All of these authors, and the others too, must have found a way to discount the First Law of Thermodynamics in order to venture their hypothesis that calories don't count. Newton would roll over in his grave.

I agree with the critics who attack the calories-don't-count aspect of the low-carbohydrate diet: Calories Do Count, they always have Counted; they always will Count. There's no metabolic advantage to the low-carbohydrate diet in **wasting** energy. As I've shown, there's a metabolic advantage to the diet only in the fact that it drives fuel into the active tissues for burning thereby **reducing food intake**. The high-carbohydrate diet, in contrast, induces, as we've seen, the conversion of glucose into fat, a mechanism little discussed by most in the scientific community.

Weight Loss, Appetite, and Hunger

With **calorie intake controlled**, the low-carbohydrate diet leads to the loss of more **bodyweight** compared with the high-carbohydrate diet, in the short-term. Proponents claim that this increased bodyweight loss is composed of fat and, therefore, they claim, one loses more fat on a low-carbohydrate diet than when following a high-carbohydrate diet. This is true, to a small degree, as I've shown. Yet, the proponents ignore that **most** of this increased bodyweight loss is a function of water losses. By ignoring this fact, they hype this diet to their marketing advantage: It's best to keep the public in the dark when selling your product, or so they seem to imply.

Bodyweight loss, however, is **not** the critical feature in looking good, fat loss and changes in body composition are. I've established that the low-carbohydrate diet leads to somewhat higher losses of fat than a high-carbohydrate diet, but these fat losses are OK but not miraculous.

In the early weeks of a low-carbohydrate diet, however, most of the bodyweight loss is a function of water losses. The low-carbohydrate diet also decreases losses in, maintains, or increases, muscle mass, depending on calorie intake. If one uses the low-carbohydrate diet for a long time, he will lose more fat and maintain more muscle than one who follows a high-carbohydrate diet. But these differences rarely amount to more than about a 10 pound swing in each.

In other words, the long-time low-carbohydrate diet follower may have 10 pounds less fat and 10 pounds more lean (maximum) on his body than one who had followed a high-carbohydrate diet for a long time. This will certainly lead to a nice difference in appearance. Of course, none of this will occur if the low-carbohydrate eater is not aware of the calories he consumes.

One can consciously count calories or not count them, surrendering food intake to the unconscious controls of appetite and hunger. Most often this is the route people follow, leaving it up to nature. This is the wrong choice. Unfortunately, most low-carbohydrate proponents don't believe in calories. Many believe that counting calories is too demanding. You don't have much choice, however, if you want to control weight.

The reduction in **hunger** and **appetite**, an attribute of the low-carbohydrate diet, and the subsequent reduction in calorie intake -- plus the delivery of fuel to the active tissues and away from fat storage -- are the primary factors leading to more body fat reduction than experienced with the hunger-increasing carbohydrate-to-fat-storing low-fat diet.

The Nutrition Council's Complaints

Next, the Council outlined the potential hazards of the low-carbohydrate diet. The first, of course, is its view as to the diet's effect on blood fats: in the Council's view, the diet's gravest danger. The Council drags out the claim that high blood cholesterol and high blood triglycerides are associated with an increased risk of developing heart disease. It contends that a diet rich in cholesterol and saturated fat could be responsible for accelerating arteriosclerosis, although there's no evidence that eating meat and fat raises these blood fats. These claims have all been fabricated by the use of false data, ruthlessly misused statistical analyses, and the desire of so many to reap huge profits by continuing to maintain this dietary charade. (See Chapter 6 from my 600-page UDS for a complete analysis about the hoax that fat and cholesterol cause heart disease.)

The Council avoids any discussion of carbohydrate-to-fat conversion (I'm sure they don't even know about it) and any discussion of how the body converts carbohydrates into saturated (human) animal fat. They certainly dig themselves into a hole with this one.

It also claims that this ketone-producing diet may cause an increase in uric acid concentration, resulting, it says, in an increased risk of gout.

Next, is the claim that the low-carbohydrate diet leads to fatigue after two days. The Council says, "This complaint was characterized by a feeling of physical lack of energy brought on by physical activity. The subjects all felt that they did not have sufficient energy to continue normal activity after the third day. This fatigue promptly disappeared after the addition of carbohydrate to the diet."

Postural hypotension (dizziness upon rapidly standing) is another potential hazard in the Council's view.

Saturated Fats, Cholesterol, Triglycerides, and Coronary Heart Disease

Again, the failure of the Council to study thoroughly the literature of nutritional science accounts for its gross misunderstanding of the facts. In UDS "Big," I thoroughly discuss the idea that fat and cholesterol do not cause heart disease. All this is a result of the Council's having bought the "Establishment's" cause of heart disease. Hell, it is, after all, the "Establishment."

Here are the facts about the low-carbohydrate diet. If the Council had ever studied the diet it would have discovered that this regimen, most often, decreases cholesterol and triglycerides. It's rare that cholesterol actually rises. And triglycerides are manufactured from carbohydrates in the liver. (If there are no carbohydrates, there is low triglycerides.) Then, the triglycerides are released from the liver into the blood for transport to the fat cells for storage. In the most precise sense, carbohydrates raise triglycerides, not fat.

Ketosis

Another false fear about low-carbohydrate diets is ketosis. You can prevent ketosis by eating as little as 100 grams of carbohydrate each day. However, even if you do go into ketosis, there's no harm from it, only benefit. I know that most health practitioners will tell you that ketones are harmful, but that's true only if you are diabetic.

We must distinguish **pathological** ketosis from **physiological** ketosis. In the former, high levels of ketones are dangerous. In the latter, occurring as it does with a very low-carbohydrate intake or fasting and starvation, the regulatory mechanisms in normal, healthy people control the rise of ketones. Ketones are, after all, important to the body's fuel economy. The release of free fatty acids from the body's fat cells into the blood increases in starvation or in low-carbohydrate diets. The body, however, doesn't allow these free fatty acids to rise to dangerously high levels, preventing this by the liver's conversion of them to ketones.

As D.H. Williamson and R. Hems point out in their 1970 article on ketones, published in <u>Essays in Cell Metabolism</u>, page 257, "It is perhaps unfortunate that ketone bodies were first discovered in the urine of diabetics because this led to the natural conclusion that they were useless products of metabolism, a view which is still held by a number of biochemists and clinicians."

This view is still held by most physicians and scientists in the year 2002.

Therefore, as long as you are healthy and don't suffer from diabetes, ketosis is nothing to fret about. If you have a concern, have your physician review the large number of research papers. They'll confirm everything I've said.

Initially, when beginning a low-carbohydrate diet, there is some ketone loss in the urine. This accounts for 50-100 calories a day. After several weeks of adaptation to the low-carbohydrate diet, ketones become a primary fuel for the brain, central nervous system, organs, and muscles. This increased burning of ketones decreases their amount in the urine. In fact, after a month or two on an extremely low-carbohydrate diet, it's virtually impossible to detect ketones in the urine. They've all been burned in the cells as a source of fuel.

The critics of the low-carbohydrate diet are <u>wrong</u> when they claim that ketones are unhealthy and Atkins is <u>wrong</u> when he claims that ketones are a significant source of energy "wasting" that confers a metabolic advantage to the low-carbohydrate diet.

Uric Acid

Dr. Wolfgang Lutz, a medical doctor who used a low-carbohydrate diet in his medical practice for over 40 years, has shown that, in most people, uric acid decreases when they follow the low-carbohydrate diet. He points out, however, that there's a small subset of people in whom uric acid may increase. He believes that the people in this subset most likely have some sort of metabolic abnormality and, hence, should be evaluated medically. It may also be necessary for the people in this subset to avoid the low-carbohydrate diet or to determine how far they can pursue the low-carbohydrate diet before experiencing the rise in uric acid.

Fatigue

I absolutely agree with the Council concerning the issue of fatigue and exhaustion, but only during the first 3-14 days. It's a temporary effect, vanishing after the body adapts to the diet. One can avoid it altogether by following the right version of the low-carbohydrate diet, the Ellis version.

These symptoms are, however, self-limiting, a fact that the Council members would be aware of if they had ever tried the low-carbohydrate diet. If one has no experience in something, how can he qualify as an expert witness?

Under the influence of a high-carbohydrate diet, the enzymes that process fatty acids and ketones decrease, and the enzymes for processing carbohydrates increase. Carbohydrates increase both the enzymes that process carbohydrate as fuel and the enzymes involved in converting carbohydrate to fat.

Removal of carbohydrate from a carbohydrate eater's diet leads to fatigue. In the short term, replacement of carbohydrate by fat doesn't help relieve the fatigue. Even when fat fuel is **available** during the early days of a low-carbohydrate diet, the body can't **process** the fat. The fat-processing enzymes, long dormant, can't break down the fat arriving from both the diet and the fatty acids released from the body's fat stores because there are too few enzymes to do the job.

Dizziness

The dizziness associated with postural hypotension (standing rapidly from a seated or lying position) occurs because of the decreased supply of fuel to the brain, and the loss of water that contributes to a slightly reduced blood volume. Again, this "symptom" straightens itself out shortly. Scientific studies into fuel use by the brain have shown that, after 12 days of starvation, 75% of the brain's and central nervous system's energy comes from ketones. This adaptation, of course, also occurs in response to a low-carbohydrate diet. The biochemical and physiological changes occurring in the body are similar whether functions of starvation, low-carbohydrate eating, or exercise. Again, however, following the proper version of a low-carbohydrate diet permits one to escape this symptom of dizziness altogether.

Obesity: Diet Composition

The Council argues that fats, not carbohydrates, are the types of foods that fatten people. This, however, isn't true, as we've learned. It questions the "metabolic advantage" described by Dr. Atkins. I can state now, however, that both the Council and Atkins are wrong.

The Council published its position paper in 1973. I've discussed the fact that the earliest understanding of carbohydrate-to-fat conversion dates back to 1852. A great deal of work had already been published in the 1940's and in the 1950's about carbohydrate-to-fat conversions, long before the Council's 1973 publication. In the previous chapters, I've covered this subject of carbohydrate-to-fat conversion in detail.

They also have developed the argument that fat is the most concentrated source of calories available. This is true. The thought is that eating fat instead of carbohydrate increases calorie intake leading to obesity. Seems logical enough, doesn't it?

But...

Remember, for review, fats have 9 calories per gram and carbohydrates have only 4 calories per gram. But as it turned out, these "Council guys" made the very same interpretive mistake that other scientists had made and still make today. Here's their mistake, then, and today: They assume that people eat for food weight. In other words, if one were to cut out 200 grams of carbohydrate, these scientists argue that the individual would replace the eliminated carbohydrate by exactly the same number of grams (weight) of fat, 200. This is absolutely untrue.

The number of calories burned in the active tissues drives food intake, not the ingestion of a specific number of grams of food. More burning of food leads to less food consumption. More storage of food as fat leads to increased food consumption. Carbohydrate ingestion increases fat storage, thereby increasing food consumption. The Council guys had this one all wrong.

Eggs

The Council, in conflict with Atkins, suggests that egg yolks cause an undesirable increase in cholesterol. In 2002, this idea has become a part of the public consciousness, as witnessed by the millions of egg white omelets consumed every day by average Americans.

The Council suggests that egg yolks increase cholesterol, even though there has never been a study showing that eggs increase cholesterol. They don't. Again, this orchestrated hatred of the "perfect protein food" -- the egg -- is the product of a failure to obtain the facts, a failure to do the required research for truth-seeking, as opposed to the easy relapse into dogma.

Crushing the Criticism Against the Low-Carbohydrate Diet

The Council Bangs the Gavel

The Council concluded that the low-carbohydrate diet is without scientific merit. It is surely **correct** to dismiss certain recommendations provided by those authors promoting the low-carbohydrate diet. But it is profoundly **incorrect** about some of its other conclusions and recommendations.

The Council calls the low-carbohydrate diet a bizarre dietary regimen. I, on the other hand, see the typical American diet as the bizarre regimen. It's well known that our primitive ancestors consumed largely meat-based diets. The high-carbohydrate, high sugar diets of the modern world aren't the dietary norm that undergirds our evolution.

The Council's doctors attempt to make the low-carbohydrate diet bizarre by claiming that it is. They want the diet to be perceived as bizarre because it conflicts with their long-standing beliefs. They embark upon limited research and form half-truths that serve as the basis of their claims. Making claims for the sake of making claims proves nothing. Does the act of saying that something is the truth make it the truth? The Council's doctors expect us to believe whatever they say since they've come to be perceived by the media as the "experts."

Correcting the Errors -- On Both Sides

Again, people on **both** sides of the argument over the low-carbohydrate diet are wrong about some things and right about others. Without doubt, the "Establishment" experts are correct in disdaining those low-carbohydrate supporters holding the notion that calories don't count. The proposal by many supporters of the low-carbohydrate diet that calories don't count is, of course, the main shortfall in their program. The fact that they have missed the *primacy* of calories is astonishing. I explain how this has happened in Chapter 21 of UDS, available as an e-chapter on my site or in UDS Big.

Total calorie intake vs. total calorie expenditure determines bodyweight, and you've already learned these details in earlier chapters. No more elaboration is required now; it's been all laid-out. The "Establishment" is right on this point, and Atkins is wrong. So are all the others who say that calories don't count.

Many of the problems associated with this diet and attacked by the "Establishment" are purely a function of reducing carbohydrate intake too soon and by too much. My version of the low-carbohydrate diet corrects all these problems. I provide you with the details of my plan in another chapter later in this book.

As I've shown, the body adapts to burning the fuels it eats. The body prefers to burn fat rather than carbohydrate. In the absence of carbohydrates, fat becomes the primary fuel, but the enzymes required to process fat aren't available in the right quantity at the start of carbohydrate reduction. It takes several weeks, even several months, for the body to make a complete *adaptation* to processing fat as fuel. The "Establishment," in opposing this diet, unmasks itself as having no experience with the low-carbohydrate diet, as having never tried it or studied the scientific literature about it.

Kidney Harm

Not **one** scientific study shows that a high-protein/low-carbohydrate diet harms the kidneys. I have searched the scientific literature all the way back into the 1920's and have never found any paper showing that protein harms the kidneys. Dr. Peter Lemon, a high-protein-intake advocate for athletes, has never having unearthed any research which indicates that high-protein intakes damage the kidneys. Dr. David Kronfeld has shown that dogs who already have damaged kidneys aren't further damaged after four years of an extremely high intake of protein. Forget it, the claim of kidney damage does not stand.

Summary

In summary, people on either side of the good and the bad of low-carbohydrate dieting are both partly wrong and partly right. After almost 200 years of low-carbohydrate use, few people have put together all the evidence. But, here, I have. To reach my own personal goals, I had to do it. This book is the product of a 43-year-long campaign to unravel the mysteries of weight loss and weight control.

You'll discover that my version is effective, providing more flexibility than the Atkins version. Combined with my other recommendations, which I'll share with you in another chapter, my program is a world-class winner. There's nothing to match it. All other programs, and I do mean **all**, provide only a small portion of the total weight loss and weight control equation. They're riddled with half-truths and misinformation.

I'm telling you the whole story and the whole truth of how to lose weight and maintain that weight loss.

Chapter 12

Completing My Understanding of the Energy Balance Equation

I was eager, after my diet and work-out hiatus due to the pursuit of my Ph. D. during the 1980's, to begin systematic experimentation with my diet, so in the Spring of 1990, I decided to experiment with the low-carbohydrate diet, experimenting first with the Atkins version. As I've already noted, I promptly gained 5 pounds on this diet. I knew, however, from my detailed studies of fuel metabolism for my Ph. D., that a low-carbohydrate diet was the best way to go. I knew this not only because of my research, but also because of my experience using this diet during the late 1960's.

In those early years I hadn't yet defined the low-carbohydrate diet as such, but had drifted into it because of my desire to consume large amounts of protein. Purely by happenstance, I'd reduced my intake of carbohydrates and derived great benefit from this regimen. I'd never, however, imprinted the details of the diet into my brain because I had no idea as to what I was doing or why it worked. It just did. Any benefit that I derived from this diet came about, I thought, solely because of the high protein intake and not because of the absence of carbohydrates which would, as I came to learn, alter my metabolic machinery for the better.

Because of my failure to lose weight on the Atkins version of the low-carbohydrate diet (because, indeed, of my weight gain on it), I began to explore the biochemistry underlying a restricted-carbohydrate diet. I already understood, at that time, most of the biochemistry related to the body's processing of glucose and fat, but I knew little about an important part of fat metabolism: the part that concerned itself with the production and

Completing My Understanding of the Energy Balance Equation

use of ketones. I, therefore, directed myself toward understanding this aspect of fuel metabolism.

Dr. J. Denis McGarry and his colleague, Dr. Daniel Foster have spent their careers unraveling the relationship between, and the metabolic controls of, the body's uses of metabolic fuels. The most important review article that I found was their 1980 publication that summarized their work in coming to an understanding of the relationship between carbohydrate and fat metabolism. The only pieces of this relationship they hadn't yet uncovered related to the genetics behind the relationship. That work is now, with the advent of the new millennium, just beginning to take shape.

After reading, multiple times, and thoroughly understanding their review article (outlining it in fact in my word processor), I was now prepared to uncover the reasons for the "failure" of the Atkins diet to effect weight loss in me and in the others who also failed to lose weight or to lose as much as they wanted.

Atkins' two main claims were that 1) one could eat as much food as he liked as long as he restricted carbohydrates and 2) that the low-carbohydrate diet leads to some type of metabolic advantage in "wasting" calories. The outgrowth of his first claim was what Atkins calls the "Calorie Myth," a claim that argues that the "Establishment's" calorie theory of bodyweight control is a mistake.

I collected all the research papers that Atkins used to support his claims, and all those that he damned for refuting his claims. By this time, I knew that calories were of importance in weight control but had not yet incorporated a sense of their overarching importance into my weight control paradigm. Atkins, of course, was not the originator of the notion that, as long as one restricts his carbohydrate intake, he can consume as much food as he wants. This idea was promulgated several decades before the 1972 publication of Atkins' first book.

After I learned about ketones, it was clear to me that Atkins had, at most, achieved a rudimentary and fragmented understanding of fuel metabolism, particularly ketone metabolism. This fundamental lack of understanding seems to have led him into many misinterpretations of the science behind the diet, misinterpretations that undermined the overall effectiveness of his highly advertised low-carbohydrate protocol.

●●●●●●●●●●●●●●●●●●●●●●●●●●●

The Eskimo Diet and Vilhjalmur Stefansson

For many years I had seen references to the work of Vilhjalmur Stefansson, the renowned Arctic explorer, and his vigorous support of the Eskimo Diet. This diet, of course, was extremely low in carbohydrate and high in meat -- a true high-protein, high-fat diet. I found a copy of Stefansson's 1959 book, the <u>Fat of the Land</u> among the titles held by the Philadelphia Free Library. I went to the library, plopped myself into a high-back chair and started to read. When I got home, I scanned the yellow pages until I'd found a bookseller for out-of-print books, needing this book for my own personal library. I couldn't wait to digest Stefansson's observations about the ten years he lived with The Eskimos at the turn of the 20th century.

Stefansson adopted the Eskimo lifestyle, including their dietary patterns, while living with them in the far North. He found their diet healthful and nourishing, so much so that he was an advocate for the health value of the Eskimo-type diet for the next 40 years. He was met mostly with ridicule from many quarters throughout those decades, but did find some support from both professional and lay readers.

Completing My Understanding of the Energy Balance Equation

My Own Experiments with the Eskimo/All-Meat Diet

From all of my reading and studies, above, I finally and clearly understood where Atkins had gone wrong: Calories Do Count. One can not eat as much as he wants, and there's no "metabolic advantage" in "wasting calories" through ketone excretion, as Atkins claims. And so, finally, by 1991, I knew what I had to do: restrict carbohydrates **and** watch how much I ate. That was all there was to the dietary part of weight control.

I began a properly implemented low-carbohydrate diet -- the beginnings of the Ellis Version. I understood from my extensive readings that the initial fatigue and loss of energy when following a low-carbohydrate diet were short-lived phenomena, occurring between days 3-8, after which they vanished as quickly as they had arrived (the usual arrival day for fatigue is around day three). After several weeks on the diet, it was as though I had walked into another dimension: the experience of heightened energy and mental clarity was beyond anything I'd ever known.

All the other aspects of my health improved as well: my skin had a new sheen to it, my gastrointestinal function was excellent, my strength and obviously my endurance had improved, and I slept much better: I had a profound sense of well-being and calmness. This sense (of well-being), is one of the claims made by vegetarians concerning the vegetarian diet. I, however, had followed that diet for three years and experienced nothing but jitteriness and hunger, accompanied by fatigue and a loss of muscle. So it was absolutely amazing to me to experience these incredible changes as the function of a diet that was as different from vegetarianism as it could be.

The Caltrac

Scientists have always been interested in the problem of overweight and obesity. The Energy Balance Equation was well established by the late 1800's. Since that time, researchers had been committed to the development of methods to accurately determine what people ate, the number of calories they burned, and how these two actions were reflected in bodyweight and body composition. Many of the sophisticated laboratory methods that were developed to measure calorie burning, however, were not suitable to such measurements in free-living individuals, people outside the laboratory setting. And the human nature of human beings' "all-too-human" behavior often interfered with a thorough understanding of some laboratory findings: this made the measurements and prediction of an individual's calorie burn difficult.

Through the 1950's and 1960's, the method of choice for determining calories consumed and calories burned was a questionnaire: researchers questioned subjects about the food they normally ate and their usual physical activity. Another method of determining calories eaten and burned was a food and physical activity diary that was completed by the subject. These methods were, of course, fraught with many sources of error that made it difficult to achieve some of the most basic insights into the weight loss and weight control equation.

As the decades passed, however, increasingly sophisticated laboratory and field methods were developed for the assessment of calorie consumption and calorie burning.

In the 1960's Dr. Henry Montoye of the University of Wisconsin, who had been instrumental in developing physical activity questionnaires, began work on developing a human motion sensor.

Completing My Understanding of the Energy Balance Equation

In the early 1980's, Hemokinetics, a Madison, Wisconsin, engineering firm, purchased the rights to Montoye's human motion sensor and developed it for commercial use. Hemokinetics named the product Caltrac.

Since the scientific community was interested in the Caltrac to measure human calorie burn, many universities purchased it, conducting scientific studies on its accuracy.

Having followed the scientific work published on the Caltrac as an excellent tool to facilitate weight loss and weight control, I convinced my business partners to purchase the marketing rights for it. Our two companies came to an agreement and quickly concluded the business deal.

Thus began my task of redeveloping the Caltrac for commercial use, a process I began in 1991 and completed with the first sale of the updated version in May, 1993.

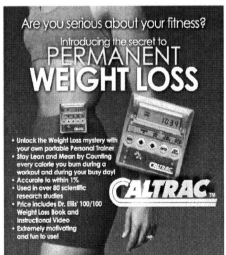

By the time we had purchased the rights to the Caltrac, more than 75 scientific papers had been published about it. It had been proved to be an accurate device for measuring human calorie burn.

The Final "Imprinting" of the Energy Balance Equation

Caltrac was, and is, the best tool ever developed for measuring calorie burn outside the laboratory. It was the tool that had been awaited for over a century of scientific research into human calorie balance. It was the tool that would make it possible for people to control their weight through an understanding, and now a measurement of, the Energy Balance Equation. Scientists needed two accurate tools to determine calorie balance: a measurement of food intake and a measurement of calorie burn. Obviously, the measurement of human food intake was very difficult unless the subject was locked into a metabolic ward. The Caltrac, on the other hand, provided a very effective method for determining calorie burn in free-living individuals.

There were, however, still errors in the calculation of calorie burn because the Caltrac is a motion sensor and cannot easily pick up movements such as fidgeting. Because one attaches the Caltrac to a waistband or a belt, the body must move for the Caltrac to sense that movement. To this end, the Caltrac is well suited to measure "relative" calorie burn rather than "absolute" calorie burn. "Relative," in this case, means that if one wears the Caltrac for a week and records a calorie burn of 3,000 daily calories and then changes his pattern, increasing his calorie burn to 4,000 daily calories, the Caltrac will pick up the additional 1,000 calories. Absolute calorie burn means that one actually burns 3,000 calories, even though the Caltrac may "record" only 2,900 of these 3,000 calories.

Nonetheless, many scientific studies show that the Caltrac does a very good job at predicting the actual or "absolute" calorie burn of an individual. Statistical correlation coefficients are often above 0.90, an excellent relationship.

Completing My Understanding of the Energy Balance Equation

At the end of 1993, I had mastered the subject of human metabolism and had come to an understanding of the Energy Balance Equation, arriving in this process to an understanding of the solution to overweight and obesity. I had also come to an understanding of the way the body metabolizes food to produce energy (and also how food is stored as fat).

By that time, I understood the fatal mistakes that Dr. Atkins had made in designing his version of the low-carbohydrate diet. The low-carbohydrate diet is effective, but the Atkins version is often not: people often quit the low-carbohydrate protocol after failing on his version. It's also important to correct his dumbing-down of the scientific facts of the Energy Balance Equation, having replaced them with his wholly un-scientific claim that "calories don't count."

I want to make sure that we separate Atkins' name from its tight association with the low-carbohydrate diet, as if he were its inventor and that his "method" of doing it, "doing Atkins" as he calls it, is the only way to use the low-carbohydrate tool. People hear of my dietary recommendations and always say: "Oh, is it like the Atkins diet?" His name has become synonymous with this diet, and his popularity is such that I can't let stand the errors that affect the bodyweight, and lives, of millions of people. My complete Atkins analysis is available on my web site or in the 600-page weight loss encyclopedia, **Ultimate Diet Secrets**. Please remember that you are reading **Ultimate Diet Secrets Lite**, the **HOW TO** version of my book with my complete **STORY** and most of the **WHYS** removed. Let's now examine the Energy-Out part of weight control, physical activity.

Chapter 13

The Importance of Physical Activity to Bodyweight Control

The Ellis System is the best innovation in the weight control business -- ever. Why? Because scientists agree: The key to weight control is balancing the number of calories you eat against the number you burn. It's that simple!

This is the **Energy Balance Equation**. As you now know, the Energy Balance Equation has two sides: **Energy-In** (how many calories you eat) and **Energy-Out** (how many calories you burn).

Considering the **Energy-In** side, there are three rules. **First**, *eating* more calories *than you burn* causes you to gain weight and get fatter. **Second**, *eating* fewer calories *than you burn* causes you to lose weight and become leaner. And **third**, *eating* the same number of calories *as you burn* causes you to stay the same weight.

The Energy-In side of the Equation is the one that most people emphasize when setting out to lose weight. They eat fewer calories.

This isn't the best choice. Let's look again at the Energy Balance Equation. But this time, let's consider the **Energy-Out** side, and look at the same three rules above, except now we'll switch the words, exchanging **burning** for **eating**. **First**, **burning** fewer calories *than you eat* causes you to gain weight and get fatter. **Second**, **burning** more calories *than you eat* causes you to lose weight and become leaner. And **third**, **burning** the same number of calories *as you eat* causes you to stay the same weight.

The Importance of Physical Activity to Bodyweight Control

Why did I switch the words **eating** and **burning**? I want to change your thinking away from the idea that losing and controlling bodyweight by the use of cutting calories is the best means towards the idea that burning more calories to lose and control bodyweight is the best means.

I'm not opposed to dieting, but it's not the most effective way to control bodyweight. And it creates problems, such as slowing your metabolism and your calorie burn.

Do Physical Activity and Exercise Contribute to Reducing Bodyweight and Body Fat?

The answer to the question above seems obvious; you must wonder why I'm even bringing it up. The answer to this question, however, is subject to so much argument that scientists still haven't concluded whether the answer is yes or no. Let's find out why there's so much argument and confusion.

Most treatment programs for overweight and obesity **assume** that exercise is a valuable addition to a weight control program. This concept, however, hasn't been critically examined. Several recent review articles about whether exercise helps in obesity appeared in the year 2000. In fact, in 1999, the American College of Sports Medicine conducted a scientific roundtable on the role of physical activity in the prevention and treatment of obesity.

The roundtable consensus certainly supports the Energy Balance Equation: One must burn more calories than he eats to lose weight. Its participants noted that energy dense foods, served in large portions, drive people's high calorie intakes. Remember, "energy dense" refers to food that has lots of calories per gram of weight.

The roundtable participants called attention to the historical fact that physical activity, both as work and as leisure, has declined profoundly for people living today, leading inevitably to the reduction in their calorie burning.

The Roundtable's Conclusions and Other Reviewers Put in Their Two Cents

And what were the conclusions from this roundtable meeting? They wrote, "Increments in energy expenditure brought about by moderate exercise are insufficient to completely forestall weight gain with advancing age or to reverse higher levels of overweight and obesity." They also concluded that current lifestyle trends in society are counter-productive to increasing calorie burning as a function of increased physical activity.

Doesn't sound too good for my old friend exercise does it?

In a 2000 review article, another reviewer states that "much data suggest that exercise does little to aid the weight loss process without the addition of some degree of caloric restriction."

This reviewer's summation was that **combining** exercise with a reduced calorie intake has little, if any, further effect on weight loss beyond that of a reduced calorie intake by itself. This is certainly counter to what most people believe, isn't it.

That's right, that's what he said: "little, if any further effect accompanied by the combination of exercise with calorie cutting." Boy, where do we go from here? If exercise doesn't help to increase weight loss, then why the hell should anybody exercise?

The Importance of Physical Activity to Bodyweight Control

Dr. Dale Schoeller said that the amount of exercise that is practical for most people to do each day adds nothing to the effect of diet alone. What does he mean "practical?" I interpret this to mean that the amount of exercise people are **willing** to do isn't compatible with the amount of exercise people **need** to do to lose weight.

Hmm... this is a problem.

Low Levels of Physical Activity Contribute to Overweight

One review article states that low levels of physical activity are linked with overweight and obesity. Another scientist says that studies consistently show that high levels of physical activity **prevent** obesity. Please note his use of the words "high levels."

There's also an important relationship between eating behavior and physical activity. I'll discuss this subject in detail soon.

The nitty-gritty of this situation, then, is that there's confusion among scientists about the value of exercise in weight loss and weight control.

In 1995, Jack Wilmore, Ph. D., a leading exercise physiologist, concluded that "formal physical activity in the form of exercise training results in relatively small changes in body mass and composition over short periods of days or weeks. This is <u>inconsistent</u> with **expectations** (emphasis mine) because physical activity constitutes a major source of daily energy expenditure." He also concluded, as do many other researchers, that in almost all cases weight loss is best achieved by combining dietary intervention with increased amounts of physical activity. His opinion as to the combination of exercise and diet and its positive impact upon weight loss conflicts, obviously, with the opinion of Dr. Schoeller, above.

Interestingly, in spite of his conclusions that exercise, by itself, is not effective in weight control, Dr. Wilmore opened his review article by discussing the effect of exercise on weight loss and weight control. The studies that he discussed in the introduction of his paper, however, demonstrated profoundly powerful results from exercise on weight loss and control. There seems to be some conflict here among the different studies.

Here are the studies he described. In two recent scientific studies, researchers demonstrated the power of calorie burning through physical activity for weight loss. These studies prove that one can lose enormous amounts of weight and fat *from exercise alone*. In a study by Hadjiolova, participants lost 27.3 pounds in 45 days (!) with *no change in diet*. The subjects exercised 10 hours a day and, amazingly, about 90% of the weight loss was fat tissue and 10% was Lean Body Mass. Losing weight by dieting leads to about a 33% decrease of Lean Body Mass. So, it's clear that the exercise preserved the Lean Body Mass and chewed up the Fat Mass.

In another study, Lee, et. al., showed that exercising 7 hours a day contributed to a loss of 27.5 pounds over 20 weeks. In this study, there was *no change in calorie intake*. Further, it permitted the maintenance of Lean Body Mass (muscle and organs) with losses in LBM of less than 10%. This defies the expected loss of Lean Body Mass (25% loss in Lean Body Mass) that normally occurs with weight loss as I described in the chapter on Body Composition.

Dr. Wilmore contrasted the studies above with several studies that reported little or no change in bodyweight. These were studies of subjects following the usual program of *limited* physical activity. One program used walking or running for 30 minutes, 5 days a week, and the other, lasting for one year, used brisk walking for 25 minutes a day. The subjects in the brisk walking study actually gained weight and fat over the one-year program!

So much for 25 minutes a day.

Settling the Confusion

Amazingly, Dr. Wilmore doesn't recognize the most important factor, staring him straight in the face. He dances around it, developing at least 10 reasons why exercise doesn't help with weight loss.

What's this most important factor? It's the amount of *time* that one spends exercising. You simply have to consider the studies he discussed in his very own introduction to understand this. He failed to include those long 7-10 hour a day exercise sessions in drawing his conclusions as to the value of exercise in weight loss. It's clear that he considered only the 25-30-minute studies.

Now, one can scream all day long that he doesn't have 10 hours a day to exercise, and he can't be blamed for screaming because few people have that much time available. But, of course, 10 hours of daily exercise leads to a loss of 27 pounds in 45 days.

Obviously, however, one doesn't need to perform that much exercise to lose weight. Based on the studies, above, I draw an irrefutable conclusion: the best strategy for weight loss and the maintenance of Lean Body Mass is a high level of physical activity each day.

Sure, it takes a lot of exercise, and most people won't do it, but it *can* be done. Later, I'll discuss the minimum amount of physical activity you ***must*** perform each day to control your weight. You can get-by on a lot less than 7-10 hours each day. One fact is inarguable: 3, 30-minute aerobic sessions a week won't cut it; without question, that's not enough.

If one is unable to be physically active, then he'll have to accept a low-calorie regimen for the rest of his life in order to control bodyweight because this is the only way he can avoid the weight gain that comes from decreased physical activity.

And, of course, diet changes are fraught with many problems, such as unremitting hunger and decreases in metabolism. It's unfortunate that dieting has become, for so many, the method of choice for weight control because it's virtually doomed to fail.

The best advice is: Invest at least an hour each day in physical activity at a level of effort equivalent to a well-paced walk. If you do, you can expect, by and large, to control your weight even without diet changes.

Description of the Exercise Prescription

Exercise physiologists prescribe exercise according to three criteria: intensity, duration, and frequency. An additional element in this prescription is the type of exercise performed. The two categories are aerobic exercise and anaerobic (resistance) training. Most people believe that aerobic exercise burns more calories than resistance exercise per unit time. Aerobic exercise is also thought to condition the cardiovascular system more effectively than resistance exercise. Resistance exercise, on the other hand, builds muscles more effectively than aerobic exercise. Further, there's a point between the two ends of this continuum where muscle building and cardiovascular conditioning overlap: a point where they occur simultaneously.

The Importance of Physical Activity to Bodyweight Control

For example, let's take walking, a purely aerobic exercise. Aerobic means that the body's calories combine with the oxygen one breathes to produce energy. (Oxygen combines with the food one eats allowing the body to "burn" it in order to provide the calories one needs.) The body doesn't need to rely on any stored energy sources in the performance of aerobic exercise. In contrast, the 100-meter sprint uses mostly the muscle's stored energy to meet calorie needs.

If, however, I load you with a 40-pound weight vest for your walk and send you up a hill, the exercise becomes both aerobic and resistance. You'll burn more calories, consume more oxygen, and build more muscle than you will by walking with no weights on a level road. Adding this load is an example of an increase in exercise ***intensity***.

I can further increase your weekly calorie burn by requiring you to do this workout seven days a week, instead of three, an increase in ***frequency***. I can pump you up even more by having you walk an hour, instead of 30 minutes, an increase in ***duration***. This is how I manipulate the three factors comprising the exercise prescription.

What's the point of all this? Generally, aerobic exercise burns more calories than resistance exercise because it's continuous instead of stop-and-go. This no longer holds true, however, if one decreases the rest period between the execution of sets in a weight training program. The intriguing feature of resistance training, as a function of its muscle building effect, is that it more dramatically changes the way your body looks than aerobic exercise. So, properly performed resistance training can increase both muscle size and cardiovascular capacity. Resistance training exercise is a better calorie burner if you lift heavy and fast: Not lifting the weight fast, but moving fast from set to set.

Physical activity exerts a powerful influence on controlling appetite and calorie intake, as we shall see. Combining the powerful controlling features of the right amount of physical activity and a low-carbohydrate diet, has a maximum effect on reducing calorie intake.

What Type of Exercise Should You Do?

The best overall physical activity and exercises are ones that involve the large muscles in your body. In the 1970's, "aerobics" became the type of exercise that was recommended most often by scientists and fitness "experts." (Aerobics is exercise whose chief characteristic is the increase in both heart and breathing rates. In a more strictly scientific definition, aerobics is exercise in which all the energy used by the body comes from mixing oxygen with food.)

Aerobic capacity is the maximum amount of work you can do using oxygen to produce energy. We measure this by a standardized test called the maximum oxygen uptake test. Scientists tell us that it's moderate physical activity, measured by total calories burned, that determines health benefits. Aerobic fitness is related to health, but the achievement of **high levels** of aerobic fitness doesn't seem necessary for optimal health benefits. Hard exercise, therefore, is not necessary to achieve good health.

Health benefits from physical activity relate to total calories burned per week. Therefore, it's unnecessary for health benefits to perform hard training in the 'target heart rate zone.' If your consultant or personal trainer promotes this idea, then you may want to look elsewhere for more "enlightened guidance."

In summary, for those who 'train-for-pain,' there is a significant difference between **health**-related exercise and **performance**-related "training." Unless you're a competitive athlete, concentrate on **duration** and **frequency**, not intensity. What counts are the total calories burned per week, not the **rate** of calorie burning.

How Exercise and Activity Affect What You Weigh and What You Eat

Why doesn't exercise get more emphasis in weight loss and weight control programs? One reason, as we've learned above, is that exercise scientists are not convinced that exercise is the weight control aid everyone believes it to be. Another reason is that most programs for weight loss and weight control concentrate on cutting calories as the main strategy. After you lose weight on your 800-1,500 calorie a day diet, what do you do when it's time to eat normally again? You do what almost everyone does: you regain all the weight you lost -- and then some.

People think that for exercise to help them control their weight that it must be long and strenuous. This isn't true. Equally untrue is the belief that small amounts of exercise or physical activity increase appetite.

Do you believe that exercise or physical activity increases appetite?

If you do, you're in for a surprise. Moderate exercise does **not** increase your appetite, and more importantly -- depending on what you do and how hard you do it -- exercise and increased physical activity might even diminish your appetite.

Many people also believe that exercise makes only a small contribution to total calorie burning. They believe that any increase in calorie burning automatically leads to an increase in food intake. In his classic 1956 study, Dr. Jean Mayer showed that human beings increase the amount they eat only in two zones: the higher end of the "Normal Activity Zone" and in the "Sedentary Zone."

This means that, at a given point in the process of increasing their daily activity, people do increase what they eat. But this usually applies only to people doing quite strenuous work over a long time.

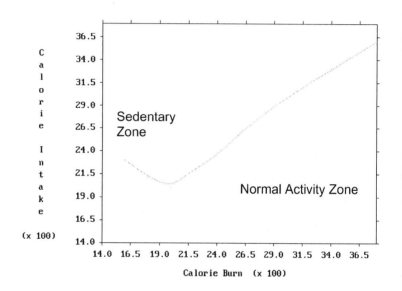

Increases in food intake automatically occur with vigorous activity to make up for the extra calorie demand. In this situation, body fat usually decreases while muscle mass increases to a point, with bodyweight remaining stable. Food intake, in short, doesn't increase enough over the long run to make one gain weight or get fatter. It increases enough only to cover the calorie burning requirement of the increased activity. This is, of course, only true in people who allow self-regulation of appetite to occur. One can easily override automatic self-

The Importance of Physical Activity to Bodyweight Control

regulation by consuming more food than required to meet energy needs. Heavyweight weightlifters are such an example.

Below the Normal Activity Zone is a zone described as the "Inactive or Sedentary Zone." This is the zone in which most people live, a zone in which one may get into trouble because of **too** little activity. In the Inactive Zone, one experiences further decreases in activity and in the calorie burn associated with activity. In this Zone, food intake often doesn't decrease and actually ***increases***. Bodyweight and body fat then increase, and muscle tissue decreases because there's too little activity to sustain it. Now, eating even a little food is actually 'too much' food because one's activity level is below the zone in which the body can ***self-regulate*** food intake.

This is the effect I expect when you follow Dr. Ellis's 100/100 Plan. Using my Plan, you'll gradually move into the Normal Activity Zone. At first, while your body re-balances itself, the increased activity isn't accompanied by an increase in appetite. This creates a Negative Energy Balance Equation leading to fat loss and muscle gain. Then, the integration of activity and a balanced intake of calories sets up a new pattern. This pattern helps you eat the number of calories you need to meet your body's requirements and to maintain a leaner and more muscular body.

If your activity level drops below the Normal Activity Zone, as it has for 60-80% of Americans, problems develop. In Mayer's study, with both human beings and laboratory animals, the balance breaks down when activity falls below a threshold level of calorie burning. When this occurs, one finds himself in the Inactive Zone.

This leads to the theory that you must do a minimum amount of physical activity before your

body can <u>automatically</u> begin to balance the food you eat with the food that you burn.

I've already discussed the studies that trace obesity to a sudden decrease in activity. Other researchers have showed this relationship between physical inactivity in children and obesity, a common research finding.

The idea of burning too few calories contrasts with what scientists and people believed years ago and still believe today: that overeating is the sole cause of the overweight and obesity problem. But, in fact, the problem of excess fat comes from too little activity. I'm sure this surprises almost everyone. It certainly underscores the idea that the majority of diet books and programs are worthless. And it must follow, then, that since almost all weight control programs are diet-based, almost all of them are worthless.

What's the Minimum Level of Physical Activity to Keep You Out of the Inactive Zone?

Recently, several researchers have re-examined Mayer's hypothesis. You must first decide how much you want to weigh and how much of that weight you want as fat and muscle. You must describe your goals.

Is your goal to get down to 15% body fat for males and 24% for females? These are sound goals. They are the ranges for college age students. After college, your weight ***can*** remain the same as it was in college. It truly can. Most people, however, lose muscle and gain fat over the 10-30 years that are subsequent to college or high school. The loss of muscle, of course, stems from a decrease in activity.

Today, I see many people, most often women, who possess normal bodyweight but, at the same time, a high level of body fat. I think our concern should shift away

The Importance of Physical Activity to Bodyweight Control

from bodyweight as the sole barometer of the "ideal." We should focus on body composition, using body composition as a barometer of our muscle-to-fat ratio. This "knowledge base" then helps us increase our muscle tissue. By the analysis of body composition we can orchestrate an exercise program that will alter our current body "style" of normal bodyweight with high fat and replace that "style" to a body "style" characterized by normal bodyweight with low body fat and high muscle. I talk more about this in my book, Dr. Ellis's **Spectrum Training System**.

How Many Calories Must We Burn to Control Bodyweight?

People burn calories at different rates depending on their body size and their level of physical activity. For our discussion, let's assume that one individual burns 15 calories a minute for a daily total of 2,160 calories. Professor E. R. Buskirk states that people stay overweight when their total daily calorie burn is in the 2,200-2,400 calorie a day level for men. For women, the range is 1,800-2,000 calories a day. He also states that, if daily calorie burn is over 4,000 calories a day, one rarely sees obesity.

If we want to observe what it takes to remain lean and muscular just look at the people who do it. Athletes provide a good example. Soldiers, in rigorous military training, provide another. Bodybuilders preparing for competition train 20-30 hours a week and eat diets containing about 2,000 calories a day, a number of calories well below their needs. As a result, they lose their body fat to make up for the difference between the calories they consume and the calories that they burn. They, essentially, eat their own body fat. We don't need more scientific studies to confirm what's already obvious to our eyes.

Dr. Gregory Ellis's Ultimate Diet Secrets Lite

Instead of questioning the overweight people about what they do and receive mis-reports, ask lean people. In this way we'll unearth the facts.

National diet surveys show that the amount of calories that men and women eat each day are in, or close to, the Inactive Zone described by Mayer. In other words, if people had maintained the level of physical activity similar to that of the people living around 1900, they would be consuming more calories than people living today. But since the physical activity level of people living today has decreased, along with their food intake, they have entered Mayer's Inactive Zone, a Zone in which physical inactivity contributes to disrupting the in-born regulation of food intake. Modern-day calorie consumption and physical activity patterns place people very close to those described by Buskirk: 1,800-2,000 for women and 2,200-2,400 for men, reflecting the low level of physical activity.

It's my hypothesis that our intake of daily calories is in the range that may lead to obesity or keep us overweight if we already are. I see only one solution: to increase the amount of daily physical activity we do. I don't see any other choice.

Since you now understand the Energy Balance Equation, you can see that there are only two ways to maintain a normal weight: 1) eat less and be hungry all the time or 2) eat the same and increase activity.

Diet plans and cutting calories have been popular for at least 40-50 years. The earliest scientific reports showing the failure of cutting calories as a means of fat loss or weight control appeared in the 1950's. Recent studies agree with these early reports: dieting doesn't work. It hasn't worked, and it won't work, now or in the future. Give dieting up!

The Importance of Physical Activity to Bodyweight Control

OK, here it is again: if you want to eat normally and if you want to be lean, you have to increase your activity enough to reach your lean goal. The leaner you want to be, the more activity you need, unless you want to back-off on the calories you eat. Though I argue that burning 100 extra calories daily by increasing physical activity is a start, it's not enough. You may not get as lean as you like doing that amount. You may have to do more to reach your goal.

Now, you have the numbers. It seems as though the Inactive Zone is about 1,800-2,000 calories a day for women and about 2,200-2,400 calories for men. Active athletes get to the 3,500-4,500-calorie-burning range per day. **Health benefits** are better when you burn about 100 calories daily through increasing physical activity, with the health benefits increasing as calorie burning climbs to 500 extra calories daily. Burning more than 500 extra calories each day doesn't provide any further increases in health benefits. But, also, burning 100 calories daily through increases in physical activity is most likely not enough, however, for weight control.

Only muscular activity can make major changes in calorie burning. You have to make a choice. If you cut calories, you'll always be hungry: a plan that always fails in the end. This failed plan will eventuate in your return to the point from which you started in your hard dieting to lose weight. Or you can invest a few extra hours each week in mild to moderate effort activity and eat normally, never feeling hungry and looking the way you want to look. It's up to you.

What matters is the total calories that you burn; it doesn't matter how you burn them, only that you do burn them.

If you keep up activity, you can expect to keep your bodyweight close to normal. Many studies show that it's possible to fit 5 days of increased activity -- 30 to 60 minutes a day -- into busy schedules. That comes to about 3-5 hours a week. This modest time commitment and the fact that it requires only moderate effort activity undercuts any reasonable argument about one's not having sufficient time and energy to exercise. It's well within anybody's physical tolerance.

Finally, the question arises: Is obesity a disease of inactivity? Or, putting it another way: Is inactivity a **cause** of obesity? Believe it or not, many scientists won't say that inactivity is a **cause** of obesity because they postulate that the obese condition arose first, causing the inactivity.

This question, however, was settled in the 1950's when Dr. Jean Mayer's classic studies showed that inactivity is not the result of obesity but that inactivity **precedes** obesity, just like energy-partitioning via carbohydrate-to-fat conversion into fat storage **precedes** overeating.

Reviewing the Modern-Day Re-Examination of the Mayer Hypothesis

Most recent evidence supports the conclusions I've stated earlier: low levels of calorie burning are the primary cause of obesity. Calorie burning in the overweight individual is greater than in those who are lean, a fact we've already established. For many years, it was believed that overweight people had a metabolic defect, that they handled calories more efficiently than normal weight persons. We now know this isn't true. This apparent paradox was settled when scientists finally realized the obvious: overweight people under-report their daily calorie intake.

Many studies show that greater weight gain occurs in adults who are inactive than in those who are active. The

The Importance of Physical Activity to Bodyweight Control

studies also show that overweight, Body Mass Index (BMI), and Fat Mass all increase as physical activity decreases.

Let's refresh your memory of a few terms. Your Total Daily Energy Expenditure (TDEE) has three parts: The first part comprises the calories you're obligated to burn each day, the Resting Metabolic Rate (RMR), which varies primarily according to changes in Lean Body Mass and, as we've seen, changes in bodyweight and reduction in calories. The second part of TDEE comprises the Thermic Effect of Food (TEF) which accounts for about 6-10% of TDEE, a figure that is so consistently constant and unvarying under many different conditions that we discount it. Physical Activity Level (PAL) comprises the total amount of calories one burns beyond RMR. Any type of physical activity is included in PAL: from Structured Exercise sessions to any type of Spontaneous Physical Activity, such as fidgeting.

Researchers measure both TDEE and RMR, subtracting RMR from TDEE to arrive at PAL. Therefore, the ratio of TDEE:RMR is PAL or the Physical Activity Level. Through extensive studies using doubly-labeled water, researchers have calculated a multiple of RMR (Resting Metabolic Rate) to determine the amount of activity that maintains a normal bodyweight.

The results of the studies indicate a threshold in PAL for maintaining normal bodyweight. In other words, PAL must reach a certain level each day if one wants to maintain a normal bodyweight. The calculated figure for determining the threshold of PAL is a multiple of RMR, which averages 1.75 X RMR. As you recall, the Total Daily Energy Expenditure (TDEE) for the typical male is 1.55 X RMR. For the typical female, it's 1.56 X RMR.

In women, a threshold of 1.75 X RMR represented the TDEE at which bodyweight stabilized, neither increasing nor decreasing. Other studies support this threshold of activity level.

Let's "put-some-numbers-to-it" in order to help make the calculations easier to understand. Assume that RMR equals 1,500 calories a day and that Total Daily Energy Expenditure (TDEE) is 1.75 X RMR. In this example, PAL equals 0.75 X TDEE. Here's the overall calculation: RMR @ 1,500 calories a day plus PAL @ 1,125 calories a day (0.75 X 1,500 = 1,125) equals a TDEE of 2,625 calories a day (RMR of 1,500 plus PAL of 1,125). The PAL part of TDEE comes from all movements during the day: both Structured Exercise and Spontaneous Physical Activity.

In this example, to maintain bodyweight, this individual must burn 1,125 calories a day beyond his RMR of 1,500 calories a day. You, I hope, performed these basic calculations for yourself in an earlier chapter. These numbers provide you with a way to "put-it-to-the-numbers," the all-powerful Ellis Method of weight loss and weight control. These calculations and your daily calorie burn subscribe to the Laws of Nature. Therefore, these calculations are guaranteed to guide you to a successful weight loss and weight control program.

Here's an example. Weight reduced, formerly-obese women whose TDEE was greater than 1.75 maintained their reduced weight. Women whose TDEE was lower than 1.75 gained weight. When the women who regained weight embarked upon an exercise program that required a TDEE at 1.75 X RMR, weight gain stopped.

How Much Physical Activity Do We Need to Lose Weight and Maintain the Loss?

It's clear, therefore, that there's general agreement among most studies regarding the amount of physical activity required to maintain a normal bodyweight. To maintain a normal Body Mass Index (BMI) and Fat Mass,

The Importance of Physical Activity to Bodyweight Control

our Total Daily Energy Expenditure (TDEE) must be at or above 1.75 X RMR. These calculations are all easy to perform. Their use grants you complete power over your bodyweight.

We know that many athletes' TDEE is between 2.0-2.5 X RMR. These athletes not only maintain a normal bodyweight but also attain low levels of body fat, often far below "normal" body fat averages.

My point in the exercises, above, is to provide you with a guide as to the required amount of exercise needed for weight maintenance. Simply making the statement, "Get some exercise," is inappropriate, providing you with no information.

Here are the final numbers. A TDEE of less than 1.55 represents light activity. Moderate activity is 1.55-1.75, and heavy is greater than 1.75. Most subjects in experimental studies whose TDEE is less than 1.75 gain weight. So, that's the level of TDEE needed.

In terms of calories, one must burn 11 calories per kilogram of bodyweight a day to maintain weight. So, divide your weight in pounds by 2.2 to arrive at kilograms. Multiply this number by 11 to figure out how many activity calories you need to burn each day. For example, if you weigh 145 pounds, divide that by 2.2 which equals 70 kilograms; 70 kilograms times 11 equals 770 physical activity calories a day. That's the total amount above your RMR that you need to burn in order to maintain a normal bodyweight.

We can place this value in perspective by converting it to a time factor. You need to perform about 75 minutes a day of moderate physical activity, such as brisk walking, to reach the required calorie burn. If you perform vigorous activity instead, your time investment is between 35-40 minutes a day.

Now, remember the average individual, just by living, burns calories at the rate of 1.55 X RMR. One needs to get to 1.75 X RMR to maintain normal weight. This requires the addition of 0.20 X RMR beyond the amount used just to stay alive and to meet the demand of moving around each day. What does this mean in calorie burning above the level necessary to sustain life and its daily activities? Let's assume an RMR of 1,500 calories a day. 1,500 times 0.20 equals 300 calories a day. That's it; that's what it takes in extra calorie burning beyond the number needed to sustain life and move around.

Other recent studies show that 1,000 calories of physical activity a week (142 calories a day) isn't sufficient to maintain weight loss. But 2,500 calories a week does maintain bodyweight. Participants enrolled in the National Weight Control Registry report successful weight loss and weight maintenance as a result of burning about 2,800 calories a week, 400 calories a day above RMR plus the calories required to move around each day (above 1.55 X RMR). My point is this: 30 minutes of moderate physical activity 3-5 times a week won't cut it.

What's the Cause of Obesity?

These results, above, confirm the influence of the environment upon increasing calorie intake and upon decreasing physical activity. In understanding the rapid increase in the Nation's obesity, we must always consider the two together. A low calorie burn wouldn't cause obesity if the body automatically adjusted its calorie intake downward to match the reduced burning rate. Unfortunately, as calorie intake has decreased during the last few decades, physical activity has decreased even further, and, therefore, intake still exceeds calorie output! It seems that our in-born ability to reduce our calorie intake depends upon physical activity that must meet a threshold level of calorie burning in order that

The Importance of Physical Activity to Bodyweight Control

food intake **automatically** regulates itself to match calorie burn and calorie consumption rates.

As a result, the most likely explanation for the high levels of obesity today is that our environment doesn't require high levels of calorie burning. The human animal hasn't evolved the capacity to reduce calorie eating to a level at which it matches the low level of calorie burning. This creates a situation in which Energy-In exceeds Energy-Out. As a result, we break the Law of the Energy Balance Equation, and overweight and obesity result.

Therefore, the onset of the Nation's obesity arises from a societal environment that celebrates eating and its pleasures while putting the brakes to activities, in nature, that burn calories. These environmental pressures disrupt our homeostasis.

The increase in an individual's Fat Mass will, eventually, level off. As bodyweight increases, so does calorie burning, primarily because of the cost of carrying the extra weight. And a new Set-Point occurs at this higher bodyweight where the higher calorie intake will once again match the increased calorie burn accruing solely from the increased body mass. Although a little confusing, calorie burning from activity is still lower today than it was years ago which contributes to overweight. Unfortunately, this new, higher Set-Point means that you will remain at this new level of fatness until you return to Nature's homeostatic balance point.

The combination of the appropriate amount of physical activity and the Ellis version of the low-carbohydrate diet are powerful allies in using Biology, instead of Willpower, to control bodyweight.

Chapter 14

What Changes Can You Expect From Increased Physical Activity?

The increase in weight that most people experience beyond age 25 (assuming they didn't get fat before that age) is the result of a large increase in body fat. Although Lean Body Mass increases with Fat Mass, there may be some loss of muscle tissue (or less Lean Body Mass increase than expected with an increase in bodyweight) as a result of decreasing physical activity.

Increasing physical activity causes changes in our body shape because we increase muscle tissue and lose fat: most people lose the accumulated fat around their waist and hips and gain muscle in the torso and extremities. These two changes -- losing fat around our middle and increasing muscle in our arms, torso, and legs -- improve our body shape.

The key concern, however, is body composition: the amount of fat and muscle you possess and the percentage they represent of your total bodyweight. Muscle and fat are the two body tissues that exercise and activity affect. It's clear, by now, that concern over total bodyweight is too simplistic because it provides little information about changes in muscle and fat.

There's good news about losing weight while exercising: You lose less muscle and more fat.

In four studies, bodyweight and body fat followed the same path with subjects becoming leaner and losing weight in response to a 9-20-week-long jogging program. In all studies except one, the exercisers maintained their Lean Body Mass, and in that one study, the exercisers actually <u>gained</u> Lean Body Mass. In another adult male

What Changes Can You Expect From Increased Physical Activity?

study lasting 2 years, the subjects dropped bodyweight by 6% and dropped body fat percent by 20% (relative, not absolute -- 20% loss of original amount).

This is exciting stuff.

The advantages of using exercise to lose and control weight are now obvious. Exercise and other types of increases in moderate effort physical activity produce losses in two ways. They

1) control or suppress appetite and
2) increase daily calorie burn, leading to an unbalanced Energy Equation that's concentrated on burning more than one takes in.

I want to remind you: You lose large amounts of Lean Body Mass when you take off weight by cutting calories as your primary method of weight control. It doesn't matter if you cut a few calories or many, but the more you cut, the more Lean Body Mass you lose. Even cutting as few as 100 calories a day contributes to a loss in bodyweight, but some of that loss is Lean Body Mass (LBM). The pattern of body composition, as a function of losses in LBM and Fat Mass, changes in response to the amount of calorie cutting, as demonstrated in the last chapter. The more one cuts calories, the greater the loss in the percentage of Lean Body Mass.

Unless you exercise.

Exercise and activity provide considerable protection against the loss of muscle tissue (and organ weight to some degree) caused by calorie cutting. Tests of exercise as a method of LBM preservation in both animals and human beings prove its reliability. When animals are weight-reduced by the same amount, with one group having lost weight by diet alone and the other by diet plus exercise, exercisers lose more fat and less LBM.

Exercise stimulates increases in the release of fat from the fat stores, and fat lost in this way is used for energy instead of valuable muscle tissues being used for this purpose. This increase in fat burning lasts beyond the actual exercise period and stimulates more burning of fat and less carbohydrate and protein. Many argue that "after-exercise" calorie burn is a significant contributor to weight loss. This amount of calorie burning is so marginal in comparison with the calories that are burned in the "doing" of the actual exercise that it doesn't lead to any metabolic miracle in fat burning.

What Type of Exercise Should You Do?

The best overall physical activity and exercises are ones that involve the large muscles in your body.

Many people talk about exercise; however, the research, as we've seen, indicates that few people exercise often enough. We now know that the health benefits provided by regular vigorous exercise are many. But an awareness of the health value provided even by mild to moderate effort physical activity, such as walking and gardening, is new: this information is just now reaching the popular press. Recent research cites the benefits of mild to moderate effort physical activity: the reduction of risk for heart disease and increases in both longevity and quality of life. These important benefits have triggered people's desire to be more active.

Aerobics is still the first choice for many people: biking, running, swimming, and rowing are popular and excellent aerobic activities. However, the first choice for most people is walking. Walking appears to provide us with the best of all worlds. Just about anyone can do it. You can do it anywhere, and though it's not hard to do, it provides wonderful health benefits.

What Changes Can You Expect From Increased Physical Activity?

I have no more to say about aerobic activity here. As we all know, books and guides about aerobics fill the shelves of bookstores anywhere.

If you choose to become a high calorie user, burning 400-500 extra physical activity calories daily, you will have to set aside specific times each day in order to reach such a goal. A walking program is an ideal choice to help you reach this goal.

Resistance Training

People have touted aerobics for three decades. But it's only during the last several years that we've begun to see scientists extol the many values of resistance training for enhancing health. Few people, scientists included, ever considered using resistance training in weight control programs. I've known about and preached its value since the early 1960's when, as a teenager, I used weights to solve my own overweight problem.

I've done extensive investigations into the body composition of men and women. In collaboration with Dr. Zeb Kendrick, Professor at Temple University in Philadelphia, and Paul Thomas, M. S., we studied over 1,000 subjects who lived different lifestyles. In our study, we put subjects into one of 7 classes, including both men and women. The groups were normal weight people, athletes doing either aerobic exercise or bodybuilding exercise, or combinations of the two. We also tested obese subjects: some performed regular exercise and others remained inactive.

Most of the exercisers trained for years, so their bodies were well conditioned. All subjects reported having a stable bodyweight for at least 1 month prior to the start of the study. The athletes all had low body fat levels. The female bodybuilders were at 13.9% body fat vs. 17.7% for aerobic exercisers. The inactive, average bodyweight female subjects were 24.6% fat, and the inactive obese females were 37.6% fat.

The most interesting finding was that of the high Lean Body Mass for the female bodybuilders. They had almost 8½ pounds more LBM than the people in the inactive normal weight group and almost 5 pounds more lean than the aerobic exercising females. This muscle increase occurred in spite of much lower fat masses. Just look at the differences:

	Bodybuilders	Hard Aerobic Exercise	Normal Inactive
LBM (lbs.)	106.0	101.3	97.5
Body Fat (lbs.)	17.2	22.0	32.0

Results from the men's study were similar. This shows how, in time, muscle mass can increase and Fat Mass can decrease in response to resistance exercise. More important are the specific effects of aerobic exercise vs. resistance training. When you compare our study with short-term studies, you clearly see the effects of a long-term commitment to resistance training programs.

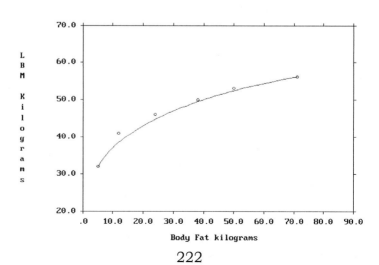

What Changes Can You Expect From Increased Physical Activity?

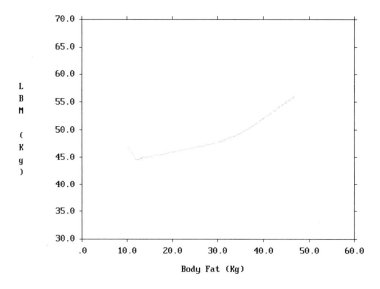

A study of the two graphs, above, shows the dramatic effect of resistance exercise in disrupting the normal relationship between Lean Body Mass loss and body fat loss that occurs with bodyweight loss. The first graph is the one previously presented in chapter 7, the chapter about Body Composition. That graph plots the data gathered by Dr. Gilbert Forbes showing that as body fat decreases, its rate of loss slows and the loss of Lean Body Mass increases.

My data, presented in the second graph, depicts what happens when one uses weight training as a primary form of exercise. You can see, that instead of losing increasing amounts of Lean Body Mass as bodyweight decreases, that this normal pattern can be reversed with one actually gaining Lean Body Mass (I'm sure as muscle tissue and not as organ tissue, although studies examining this point have not been completed). The uptick in the line in the lower graph represents the increases in Lean Body Mass occurring through weight training.

By the way, these changes only occurred with several years of training. The modern-day hypesters promising metabolic makeovers and enormous increases in muscle mass in as little as 6-12 weeks are blowing smoke at you. It cannot be done. I challenge any one of these self-professed miracle-makers to submit a study group into a scientific analysis of their claims. Do body composition tests with underwater weighing before the diet and training program begin, then at the 6-12-week points. This will take the stuff out of their balloons.

My study, along with the ones I've outlined earlier, explain how the type, intensity, frequency, and duration of exercise affect its results. The length of the training program and the number of calories cut by dieting combine to affect the changes in body composition. The message is clear, however, as to the correct way to combine training and dieting in order to achieve results:

1) The best approach to weight loss is to increase activity before you even consider cutting calories. But, you'll have to burn more than 500 calories a day to see any "happy-making" changes.
2) If the weight loss is not fast enough or the loss doesn't get you to your goal, consider cutting calories too.
3) To elevate the rate of weight loss, combine calorie cutting with exercise and other forms of increased physical activity until you achieve your weight goal. Then eat normally and sustain the level of physical activity. Work at increasing Spontaneous Physical Activity too as I'll detail in Dr. Ellis's 100/100 Plan.
4) If you cut calories, try not to cut more than 300 each day. It's probably better to level-off at 100 calories or so over a longer time to avoid losing muscle.
5) Whether or not you are controlling or losing weight, you should do a regular program of

What Changes Can You Expect From Increased Physical Activity?

resistance exercise. This recommendation is consistent with new guidelines by the American College of Sports Medicine.

Weight training maintains and increases muscle mass better than aerobic exercise.

Isn't it easier to increase your activity to a few hours a week rather than starve yourself 24 hours, 7 days a week, for months -- and, like many people, for years? Only to gain the weight back far more quickly than you lost it. And, what happens when you get your weight down by diet? You have to live with the discomfort of eating less food and experiencing constant hunger. If you can't stand the suffering, of course, you return to old eating patterns and regain the lost weight.

The idea of simply cutting calories, the basis of most programs, is tired, old, and failed. A new age is upon us, and it's up to you to take advantage of this information.

Exercise Increases Metabolic Rates: Myth's Triumph Over Truth

"Metabolic abnormality" has provided, for many decades, a catch-all explanation for people's failure to achieve weight loss. The best of current-day scientific studies prove, however, that abnormalities in metabolism are more myth than reality and are without basis in scientific fact. It's now well known that very few people have genetic or metabolic abnormalities that prevent them from losing weight.

The belief that abnormal metabolism is a root cause of obesity is deeply ingrained in our collective consciousness. It will probably prove impossible to dislodge this powerful, core-grabbing belief from most people's minds, but I'll try.

Today, the metabolism evangelists have upped the ante, proclaiming their triumphal new understandings of metabolism and its science! These new-age "experts" shout to the media, indeed to anyone who'll listen, their latest scientific gleanings from the junior varsity dietary experts and gurus who blanket the landscape of pseudo-science.

The newest "twist" actually comes directly from the fitness experts (who should know better). This theory is fodder for the marketing machine that drives an explosion of new products and programs proposed to rev-up the metabolic fires.

This new twist proclaims that adding muscle and Lean Body Mass through exercise stokes the metabolic machinery, **turning-on the engines of calorie burning even while the body is at rest!**

Adding muscle through exercise doesn't lead to a significant increase in calorie burning at rest.

Resting muscle is not active and muscle burns few calories unless it's working. There's no free lunch.

We've all been conditioned to **think** that muscle burns more calories than fat. Everyone says it, even so-called scientists. The people's "collective wisdom" about the stratospheric rise in calorie burning that accompanies increased muscle mass is an example of hearsay. It's myth having become dogma.

Muscle at rest burns few calories: it's less active than organs, which burn about 15-40 times more calories than muscle. Indeed, any large increase in muscle mass actually dilutes the increase in calorie burn that occurs when all the lean parts have increased equally in weight. There's almost no increase in organ mass from resistance exercise, including weight training. Therefore, resting metabolic rate doesn't rise as people have been taught to

What Changes Can You Expect From Increased Physical Activity?

believe when increases in muscle mass largely represent the majority of the increase in Lean Body Mass. Weight gain, therefore, occurring because of exercise, increases muscle mass while weight gain without exercise increases all components of the Lean Body Mass as well as increases in Fat Mass.

When untrained people gain weight without exercise, their muscles and their organs increase in proportion to body size. In this scenario, the organs and muscles represent the same percentage of a 250-pound man's LBM as they do in a 150-pound man's LBM. In athletes, however, most of their enhanced LBM is a function of muscle mass, which increases out of proportion with increases in organ mass.

Research shows that the metabolic activity of muscle is about 1/15th-1/40th that of organs. Therefore, I calculated the metabolic rate for the "extra" muscle in a bodybuilder based upon the research I had done on bodybuilders in my laboratory. I used the metabolic rate for muscle, not the metabolic rate for both muscle and organs, to make this calculation. The difference in total 24-hour metabolism came to only 20-50 calories for the "extra" muscle in females and 44-80 calories for males.

There has been a small amount of scientific evidence showing that activity increases a muscle's RMR, but most evidence clearly shows that there's no increase. The RMR in aerobically trained muscle is, at most, only ever-so-slightly higher than in bodybuilder's muscles. Both rates are only slightly higher than those of inactive people's muscles. Moving away from these observations, it's clear that the difference in metabolic rate, even in big males of different fat and muscle levels, is less than 100 calories a day. For a female, this metabolic rate difference is about 25 to 50 calories each day.

A change in activity, however, can increase your calorie burn by hundreds of calories daily. Likewise, if you cut calories by decreasing your food intake, you can cut hundreds of calories, up to as many as two thousand calories daily. These are the big changes: total activity, or decreasing calorie intake, that make a real impact on weight control, not more resting muscle.

What about the calorie burn during exercise? This is physics, plain and simple. The lean 200-pounder and the fat 200-pounder both move 200 pounds. The calorie burning required by that exercise is the burning of calories to move 200 pounds. That makes the calorie burning equal. It's no more complicated than that. Bodies are generally similar in their efficiency of movement. As an example, any laboratory scientist knows that, no matter what the person's body composition is, the calorie burning of riding a stationary bike is similar, regardless of bodyweight or body composition: The calorie burning of turning the flywheel is the same for each person. Although the **maximum rate** of calorie burning is different for trained and untrained people, the calorie burning at **similar** workloads is **equal**. It's just that the trained person can perform at a higher level than the untrained one before each maxes-out at their respective workloads, the workload being higher for the trained person.

The Differences in Metabolism Between Fat and Muscle

As a result of detailed analyses of organ and tissue contributions to metabolic rate, research shows that fat tissue has a low metabolic rate. Each pound of body fat possessed by an individual burns about 2 calories a day. The total daily calorie burn of all the fat possessed by an individual, who is 20% body fat, represents about 5% of the body's total daily calorie burn.

What Changes Can You Expect From Increased Physical Activity?

Although muscle is the largest tissue in the whole body, accounting for approximately 40% of an adult's bodyweight, its estimated Resting Metabolic Rate (RMR) is also low, like that of fat, at about 4.6-6.8 calories for each pound during the whole day. Because muscle tissue comprises such a large percentage of the total bodyweight, even with its low metabolic rate, the total muscle mass's contribution to total daily calorie burn is about 20-25% compared with 5% for fat, that is, of course, in an individual who is not fat.

Many people believe and say that, "Muscle burns many more calories than fat." Obviously, from these numbers, above, muscle burns 2-3 times more calories than fat (2 calories burned for each pound of fat and 4.6-6.8 calories burned for each pound of muscle during the day). It's important, at this juncture, to understand that both fat and muscle at rest are low calorie burners!

In comparing two different numbers, we must always be specific and, in this case, ask 2-3 times more than what? In this case, each pound of muscle burns about 5-6 calories compared with 2 calories for each pound of fat during the day. Fat's overall daily calorie consumption is, simply, low, not making that much contribution to the total daily calorie burn of the whole body. The calorie burn by muscle at rest is, like that of fat, also, low. Yet, by virtue of its larger contribution to total bodyweight, muscle does contribute to a more significant amount of calorie burning during the day than fat. But, the addition of several pounds of "extra" muscle through exercise, particularly weight training, will make little further contribution to total daily calorie burn because of its low resting metabolic rate. Do you see how it works, by-the-numbers?

So the apparent fat burning dynamo that resting muscle is supposed to be is just not true. At rest, muscle only burns about twice as many calories as does fat.

Let's contrast the calorie burn of fat and muscle with some of the body's organs. The liver burns 90 calories per pound of liver tissue during the day. The heart and kidneys each burn 200 calories for each pound of these two tissues during the day. Obviously, these organs don't weigh much, but all of these little teeny organs burn 60% of the body's total daily calories. Muscle, as we've seen, burns 20-25% of the body's total daily calories, far less than all of the organs combined (and muscle represents 40% of one's bodyweight).

Using a 200-pound male as an example, shows that his body has 80 pounds of muscle (40% times 200 pounds). Now, its not only "extra" muscle that burns calories, but every pound of muscle in the body as well. 40 calories per pound times 80 pounds equals 3,200 calories a day, about 1,300 more than his predicted RMR. And this is for muscle only which represents about 20-25% of the body's total daily Resting Metabolic Rate. His body fat contributes another 60 calories to this amount, so muscle and fat burn 3,260 calories a day according to the preposterous claim. Fat calorie burning is about 5% of the total calories burned per day in the body, so that muscle and fat account, then, for 30% of the total calories burned by the body each day.

The organs (brain, liver, kidneys, lungs, spleen, etc.) account for between 60-80% of the total calories burned. Let's use 70% for our calculations. The organs, therefore, would burn 10,866 calories a day. Adding this amount to those burned by muscles and fat yields an astonishingly ridiculous, unrealistic figure of total daily calorie burning of 14,126! And this is only the Resting Metabolic Rate.

Do you see how thoughtless these absurd claims are when you just take a few minutes to actually put-the-numbers-to-it? The sad tale is that every personal trainer in the country is chanting the same story.

What Changes Can You Expect From Increased Physical Activity?

Drop the myth that building muscle revs-up calorie burning!

There's another myth about metabolism, as I've said above, that circulates freely among those who think themselves knowledgeable about exercise and diet and this one is all about how exercise leads to a miraculous increase in post-exercise calorie burning that's purported to significantly contribute to bodyweight regulation. It's not true and after-exercise calorie burn makes little contribution to total daily calorie burning.

Again, I reiterate, it's muscle in motion that burns calories, not muscle sitting around doing nothing. Muscle contraction uses energy and burns calories. Muscle at rest is at rest, and burns about 5 calories per pound per day.

Chapter 15

Putting the Program Together & Dr. Ellis's 100/100 Plan

We've traveled a long road in your education about weight loss and weight control. This book, unlike any others you've ever read for information about weight loss and weight control has taught you the 100% complete weight control equation. I've convincingly established that the control of bodyweight is a function of the Laws of Nature: the Energy Balance Equation. Everyone is subject to these Laws. Everything that you do to lose and control weight must, somehow, impact upon the Energy Balance Equation. Nothing else is remotely possible.

We've learned that Metabolic Adaptations and diet composition affect and modify the straight-forward mathematical calculations of the Energy Balance Equation. Therefore, we have to make adjustments to the Energy Balance Equation when we lose weight. The Energy Balance Equation is still, however, always in operation and is the force behind weight control.

There's no other weight loss and weight control program that teaches all aspects of how to lose weight, how to maintain the losses, and what happens to a body that either loses or gains weight. Most weight loss programs have, as their basis, a diet of some kind. And, as we've seen, a diet, alone, is a poor way to attempt to control bodyweight.

Without mastering the fundamentals, I'm convinced that people believe, as I've said, that there are **hundreds**, yes, possibly even thousands, of methods to control weight. The available menus and theories about weight loss are staggering and confusing. It's a rare occurrence when I encounter individuals who actually understand

Putting the Program Together & Dr. Ellis's 100/100 Plan

the basic ideas of weight loss and weight control. People talk about "such and such diet" or "such and such exercise program," debating the merits of each. I constantly hear people exclaim that they heard that you weren't supposed to..., or you were supposed to..., (you can fill in the blanks). And, one could fill in the blank with hundreds of "plans."

I've laid-out every possible method to help one lose and control his weight. And, I've prioritized these methods to the power of their effects. Each individual can choose, according to his liking, what parts of the program he wants to follow. For example, I've emphasized the most important factor in the growing epidemic of obesity is the decreased physical activity of persons living in the modern world.

I'm realistic enough to know that most people just do not want to increase their physical activity. They don't want to join an exercise club or follow a personal exercise program; they just won't do it. People who refuse to increase their physical activity, and who want to control their weight, are then stuck with dieting as their only solution. It's not a good solution, but it seems to be the solution that most people have chosen to use for the last half-century. This may be because we've all been brainwashed to believe that dieting is the most effective solution, or it may be because no one has ever taught people about the importance of physical inactivity as the **primary** cause of overweight.

I think that people overrate dieting because of the influence of the massive number of weight loss books concentrating on diets of all sorts as the solution to weight control. Few people have ever emphasized the importance of physical activity and fewer still have provided the means of increasing physical activity other than heart-pounding structured exercise programs. I don't believe that the solution to obesity lies within structured exercise programs, just as I don't believe that it lies in dieting.

Concentrating on the Energy-In side of the Energy Balance Equation is, obviously, controlling calorie intake. If, for example, one cannot overcome his fear of fat, disagreeing with my position about diet composition, he can consume a diet composition other than my recommended low-carbohydrate diet. I've thoroughly educated my readers about the effects of diets of different compositions, so if you choose not to follow the low-carbohydrate plan then the next best choice would be a diet that is low in fat and low in energy density. All of my critics would now jump from their seats and applaud me because, with this recommendation, I join the "Establishment."

My main goal in this book is to dispel the confusion reigning over weight control. I have sought to find the facts, not caring who I piss off in the process.

Dr. Ellis's 100/100 Plan

Based on the Energy Balance Equation, I've developed the most logical, the most sensible, and the most powerful weight loss plan ever devised. This is Dr. Ellis's 100/100 Plan. What is Dr. Ellis's 100/100 Plan? I've told you that the secret to weight control is nothing more than balancing the calories you burn vs. the calories you eat. That's it! The Energy Balance Equation.

At the heart of my program to help you lose and control weight are some of the most powerful methods ever presented. One of the main goals of my program is to provide you with **Biological** controls that work as an ally to Nature's Laws. It has been my experience that the use of cognitive, or awareness controls, also called Behavior Modification, although effective, rely primarily

Putting the Program Together & Dr. Ellis's 100/100 Plan

on **Willpower**. As I have repeatedly stated, **Biology** will always win-out over **Willpower**.

My 100/100 Plan bases itself on the two parts of the Energy Balance Equation: Energy-In and Energy-Out. Each of the 100's applies to one of the two sides of the Energy Balance Equation. In using the Plan, one manipulates either, or both, sides of the 100/100 Plan to attain their weight loss goals.

For example, let's take the Plan at its face value to see exactly how it works. If one were to decrease his calorie intake by 100 calories a day and increase his calorie burn by 100 calories a day, the net change would be 200 calories a day. Using the very simplistic formula that says each pound of fat has an energy value of 3,500 calories, one would lose one pound of fat in 17½ days by following the basic 100/100 Plan. We know that the simple formulation that predicts that a pound of fat has an energy value of 3,500 calories won't hold up over time as one loses weight because of Metabolic Adaptations and because the body loses both fat and Lean Body Mass at the same time.

I've also argued that the most effective way to lose weight is through increasing calorie burn as opposed to decreasing calorie intake -- dieting. Don't cut calories by dieting but burn more by increasing physical activity. The key to the effective use of Dr. Ellis's 100/100 Plan is knowing how many calories you burn each day through physical activity. You can use a number of tools to determine daily calorie burn, such as step counting devices and charts of the calorie burning for various activities.

The most powerful measuring device, as we've seen, is Caltrac, which gives you complete control and knowledge about the Energy-Out part of your daily activities.

Why Dr. Ellis's 100/100 Plan Works Where Others Won't

You can't beat this logic: Burn 100 calories a day more than you eat and you'll lose weight (for awhile at least until Metabolic Adaptations take hold). Other 'plans' are like holding your breath. When you stop holding, you gasp for air. And when you stop dieting, your body gasps for food and demands more than you need. That's why diets fail. And remember, meeting a biological threshold of physical activity each day is an effective **Biological** control of food intake. Those who fail to reach this threshold are automatically driven to eat more food despite their reduced calorie needs!

In the second part of Dr. Ellis's 100/100 Plan, you try to eliminate 100 calories from the number of calories you normally eat each day. This way you'll get even faster results. Example: just use one less pat of butter each day.

Result? For the average female on Dr. Ellis's 100/100 Plan, a loss of 2 pounds in one month with no other changes in activity or eating habits. That's very effective and does not require that much change. Want to save more calories? Just substitute a diet soda for the regular soda that you normally drink. Save 150 calories.

Results? You'd better believe it. Just following my sensible and effective 100/100 Plan will help you lose more than 20 pounds in less than a year (using the not true 3,500 calories = one pound of fat formula). Because of Metabolic Adaptations, people always lose less weight than predicted by the simplistic formula so one must make constant adjustments if he needs to keep losing to reach a pre-defined goal. The increase in activity is just what the doctor ordered. Increasing activity each week by just walking a bit more will make you feel and look better. It will improve your health and fitness. With this plan, I take you from the old painful philosophy of "No

Pain, No Gain" to the new slogan for the 21st century of "All Gain, No Pain." It's sensible and it works!

Step by Step Approach to Using Dr. Ellis's 100/100 Plan

Run the basic calculations of Resting Metabolic Rate (RMR) and Total Daily Energy Expenditure (TDEE) for yourself that I described in an earlier chapter. Subtract RMR from TDEE to arrive at your Physical Activity Level (PAL). Remember, an average PAL for most inactive people is about 1.55 times their RMR.

Here's how to use Caltrac to make these calculations for you. Program in your personal information: height, weight, age, and sex. Wear your Caltrac during the next 5 days and calculate your own daily activity calorie burn. Make sure that 2 of these 5 days are over a weekend. You want to know your average daily activity calorie burn. You can do this for several 5-day periods if you like. However, recent research shows that one 5-day period is enough as long as it's a typical 5 days. One of the Caltrac LCD displays is for the number of calories burned as physical activity calories. At the end of the day, read the display and write the number of calories down on a piece of paper or in your weight loss diary/journal. Add up each of the five days and divide it by five to arrive at your daily average calorie burn. (Caltrac cannot account for Metabolic Adaptations other than those related to the loss of bodyweight. It can't detect decreases in calorie burning because of a reduction in calorie intake and it can't detect increases in "metabolic efficiency." You'll have to account for these as you go along.)

After following this procedure, you'll know your average daily activity burn that now serves as your baseline or reference point. (Remember, the key to success is "putting-it-to-the-numbers.") If you burned

Dr. Gregory Ellis's Ultimate Diet Secrets Lite

300, or 400, or 500 activity calories a day, and you are overweight, then, in the past, this just wasn't enough to help you get your weight down. Doing this much (or this little) each day led to your overweight condition. So, from now on, you have to do more activity or resort to calorie cutting. Your best choice is to increase your average calorie burn by 100 calories each day -- Dr. Ellis's 100/100 Plan. Then, lose (or don't gain) 1 pound that month.

How do you burn the extra 100 calories? Anyway you want!

Structured exercise. Walking a little now, a little later. Or walk the 100 calories off all at once. Dance. Garden. Clean the house (yuk!). Mow the lawn. Fly a kite. Pick-up seashells. Whatever you want is OK. Just burn 100 more.

Do you want faster results? Simply cut out 100 calories each day from what you eat -- the second 100 in Dr. Ellis's 100/100 Plan. Here's a sample list:

Food	Save
• cut out ½ bagel	85 cal.
• cut out 2 pieces thin-slice bread	110 cal.
• eat 1 orange instead of ice cream	210 cal.
• have more broccoli, no potato w/butter	195 cal.
• trim fat from steak	200 cal.
• pot roast -- eat the lean only	95 cal.
• eat 2 slices of bacon instead of 4	90 cal.
• diet soda instead of full strength one	150 cal.
• eat 2 eggs instead of 3	80 cal.
• eat 1 orange instead of 12 oz. of juice	100 cal.
• white milk instead of chocolate milk	60 cal.
• have milk instead of a milkshake	210 cal.
• eat your pizza without pepperoni	70 cal.
• slurp chicken rice soup instead of rice	50 cal.

Putting the Program Together & Dr. Ellis's 100/100 Plan

Substitutions work great. With a 100 calorie increase in activity and 100 calories saved from what you eat, you'll lose (or not gain) 2 pounds in 1 month.

Now, I want to refresh your memory about what we've learned in the chapters on the amount of physical activity required to help lose weight and maintain the weight loss. First, let's review the average TDEE currently existing in modern America. It's about 1.55 times Resting Metabolic Rate (RMR). So if RMR is 1,500 calories a day then Total Daily Energy Expenditure (TDEE) is RMR times 1.55 = 2,325 calories. Physical Activity Level (PAL) equals 2,325 (TDEE) - 1,500 (RMR) = 825 calories.

The threshold reported in scientific studies of a TDEE to maintain weight loss is about 1.75 X RMR. The math shows that the difference of 1.75 minus 1.55 is how many additional PAL calories one needs to burn each day. That's a difference of 0.2, which we multiply times your RMR of 1,500 and arrive at 300 additional PAL calories a day.

Generally, most research has shown that the typical American needs to expend 400 more calories a day beyond the 1.55 multiple of RMR to maintain their weight loss from a diet/exercise program, very close to the amount that we just calculated. Therefore, the basic 100/100 Plan may be too low. Obviously, the calculations for increases in physical activity made no provision for decreasing calorie intake whereas the 100/100 Plan does.

The 100/100 Plan provides a great amount of flexibility. I, obviously, recommend increasing calorie burn to control weight. But, many people cannot increase their calorie burn enough to lose weight at the rate that they want. Most often, when beginning to lose weight, I do recommend both a calorie reduction and an increase in physical activity as the best choice to attain a pre-defined goal weight.

Then, increase calorie intake to match energy expenditure while maintaining or increasing physical activity to maintain the new, slimmed down physique.

Remember this very important point about Metabolic Adaptations: for every pound you lose, you will need to eat 20-30 fewer calories a day to maintain the new weight. Or, conversely, you'll have to burn 20-30 more calories a day, per pound lost, to maintain the new weight. Or you can do a combination of both. It's your choice.

Do you want *even* faster results than the basic 100/100 Plan provides? You can go faster by changing either part of the Energy Balance Equation -- either the first part concerned with how much you burn, or the second part concerned with how much you eat, or you can change both sides. You can change 100/100 to 200/200. Or you can go to 300/300 or to 400/400. Or even to a 500/500 Plan. It's up to you.

500/500 is pushing it. You'll feel it. 500/500 is tough. That's a lot of exercise. For example, it's about 3-5 miles of walking each day, depending on your bodyweight. And even though all the diet people have you believe that cutting out 500 calories a day is easy, let me tell you that it isn't easy. Yet, if you follow my version of the low-carbohydrate diet, that'll help some people to automatically reduce their food intake by that amount because of the way that diet type satisfies hunger. We'll talk about it in more detail later, but the low-carbohydrate diet will, for about 50% of all people, automatically lead to a reduction in daily calorie intake by about 500 calories.

Putting the Program Together & Dr. Ellis's 100/100 Plan

At 500/500, you begin to risk losing muscle because dropping your intake by 500 calories will slow your metabolism. I know that the only way you can maintain your muscle with this much calorie cutting is to lift weights as part of your activity side. If you have been very inactive, then any type of exercise will increase muscle for a while.

I think 300/300 is a better level. This adds up to a deficit of about 5 pounds a month or 1.3 pounds a week, at least for awhile until the Adaptations set in. This is slightly higher than the ½-1 pound a week weight loss that experts recommend. **Your rate of weight loss rate will, of course, slow, as we've learned, because of Metabolic Adaptations. You'll have to make adjustments to account for this all-important factor.**

You may decide you want to pursue different numbers on each side of the Equation. Let's say 100/200 -- burning 100 more and eating 200 less. Or the other way round, 200/100 -- burning 200 more and eating 100 less. Any combination you want is OK. Keep in mind, though, that activity is the most important consideration. The research shows that increases in activity help you lose weight and keep it off.

However, we all now know that *Dieting Doesn't Work*. That's why I want you to make sure you don't cut too many calories.

After you lose the weight, keep up the activity and eat more (you were eating less to lose and now to stop losing, if you've reached a good point, you can eat a little more to attain weight maintenance at this new lower level). But, be careful, add calories back very gradually until you identify how much you can eat without regaining. And the minute you see that scale climbing, nip it in the bud and reduce the amount that you're eating. Depending on the amount and type of exercise, you may add some muscle tissue or prevent some of the loss of muscle tissue that naturally occurs with losses in bodyweight. Constant dieting and calorie cutting lower your metabolic rate. Exercise and activity maintain your metabolic rate unless you lose a lot of weight and it then drops because of that. And remember, exercise and activity do not increase your Resting Metabolic Rate. Exercise and activity are the direction in which you want to go for success.

If you follow Dr. Ellis's 100/100 Plan, you'll lose weight. One warning: many people under-report how much they eat. The average under-report is about 20%, often as high as 50%. So if you think you are eating 1,500 calories each day, you are probably eating about 1,800 calories. This is 300 calories more than you think you eat each day. If you're on a 150/150 Plan, then you just blew-it-out by under-reporting what you ate. Everything counts. Butter. One bite of bread. One Hershey Kiss is 25 calories.

EVERYTHING COUNTS.

If you don't lose, then watch out for possible under-reporting. Cut back some more. Perhaps you might choose to keep counting the same way you are, but go to a 150/450 Plan. It's still a 150/150 Plan, but I'm just tricking you in order to compensate for this little human quirk of under-reporting food intake.

Increase activity, keep eating the same amount of food you now eat, and weigh less. This is clearly the solution to the weight control problem.

Behavior Modification

The basis of Behavior Modification is to help people become consciously aware of their actions. I believe that Behavior Modification is an essential part of the weight loss and weight control equation. In essence, much of what I have taught you in this book is Behavior Modification. Behavior Modification is a powerful weapon but conscious control and **Willpower** will not overcome **Biology**.

Anyone can lose weight. Personal programs of dieting, commercial centers providing low calorie pre-packaged foods, drink mixes, pouch food, and physician-directed programs all provide low calorie plans to help people lose weight. This is the easiest part. Keeping off the lost weight is the tough part. This is where most people fail.

To lose weight, all you need to do is Unbalance the Energy Balance Equation until you lose the weight you want to lose. You can use any number of methods to Unbalance the Equation. However, to keep weight off, you need to use a different set of strategies. Eating a low calorie diet is not going to work over a lifetime.

Researchers list 4 essential steps:

1) **Decide what you want to change and set your goals. Then commit and motivate yourself to make the changes.**
2) **Initiate the changes by modifying your behavior.**
3) **Maintain the changes and constantly reinforce them.**
4) **Learn to deal, and live with, your success.**

The focus is habit change. You do this by eating less or by eating differently. You increase your physical activity. You make **gradual** changes. You do not focus on magic beliefs such as grapefruit pills or bronze wrist bracelets claiming to increase your metabolism. You start with facts, not myths -- and the main fact is the Energy Balance Equation.

The methods of behavior change can help those people who do not succeed with the simple first step of increasing activity. In fact, you may need to use behavior change methods in order to get yourself to make and keep the commitment to the first step of increased activity.

Another concept of behavior programs is to match the treatment to your own needs. I believe increased activity is the *first step* and a necessary approach that you should use. However, you may need to make changes in your diet. You have many options such as cutting calories, or using either a low-fat, low-energy density or low-carbohydrate diet. Others may respond by increasing meal frequency, drinking more fluids, or increasing dietary fiber. Use of counseling is another option. You can do this either individually or in a group.

Maintenance of Weight Loss

No matter what method you choose to get weight off, the most important step is to keep it off. The research into maintenance of weight loss is only ten years old. Attempts to increase the success rates for people trying to keep weight off focuses on three areas:

1) **Increasing physical activity -- this is the basis of my Plan.**
2) **Social support.**
3) **Relapse prevention.**

People who increase physical activity have a far greater chance for long-term success in controlling their weight.

Putting the Program Together & Dr. Ellis's 100/100 Plan

Increased activity is a **major** predictor for keeping lost weight off. People who increase physical activity have a far greater chance for long-term success in controlling their weight. Activity increase leads to a higher level of daily calorie burn, a heightened energy level, and feelings of well-being. Although activity is a **major** predictor of success, **studies show that few people follow** an increased activity program after completing a formal weight loss program.

Social support provides another way to help keep weight off. People form networks with others upon whom they can depend for encouragement in their efforts.

Relapse prevention methods teach you to expect set-backs. Then, when set-backs come, you know how to handle them. People who are successful at losing weight and at keeping it off do 4 things regularly:

1) **Increase Physical Activity**. This is the most important of the 4 factors. This supports the argument that I make for my Plan. Until recently, most diet management programs neglected physical activity. Even today, few programs place enough emphasis on it, it's the "poor relation" in weight maintenance. In Dr. Ellis's 100/100 Plan, increases in activity are crucial -- activity is the lifeblood of my Plan.
2) **Use Social Support**
3) **Trigger Motivation from Within**. You must do it for yourself. Instead of doing it simply to get into a pair of favorite jeans or to get ready for the beach season, you must do it because you want to change your life.
4) **Focus on Positive Changes**. Instead of simply looking at the bathroom scale, you are taught to add more items to your list of the things that you feel good about in yourself. These include lessening your risk for getting disease: Feeling

more energetic. Looking more positively toward calorie-burning.

We have looked at the 4 behaviors of people who keep weight off. Now, let's look at the 3 "problem spots" for people who are not successful at keeping weight off.

1) **Negative Feelings.** Emotional eating is a primary predictor of failure because people have a tough time dealing with anger, depression, and anxiety; they eat when they're under stress and when experiencing negative feelings. Learning to cope with these feelings is a must.
2) **Social Situations Which Can Be Deadly.** A demanding social life -- business lunches, parties, and get-togethers that involve food -- causes trouble. Traveling, hectic work schedules, and irregular eating patterns lead quickly to weight gain. Developing coping strategies for these situations is critical.
3) **Testing How Much You Can Get Away With.** You cheat. You eat foods that you know cause you trouble; you miss physical activity sessions.

Here are 6 steps to follow in order to lose weight and keep it off:

1) **Lose Weight Slowly.** No more than ½ to 1 pound each week. Gradual changes prevent you from feeling deprived.
2) **Reduce Calories Slowly** using a diet plan that fits your beliefs and needs: Either a balanced diet or one low in fat and energy density or low in carbohydrate: it's your choice. Most people support a diet low in fat. I support one low in carbohydrate. Find the plan for you.
3) **Gradually Increase Physical Activity.** Use a program that fits your needs: Structured or non-structured. Continuous or discontinuous, a little of each. By yourself or with others. Use

Putting the Program Together & Dr. Ellis's 100/100 Plan

recreational activities, sports, or daily living tasks to increase your calorie burn.
4) **Use Behavior Changes** to help you with your diet and activity changes. Here are 5 key behavior changes that you can make, leading to success:
   - **Self-Monitoring** to provide feedback on performance. This is where Caltrac fits in perfectly.
   - **Control** the situations that stimulate you to eat the wrong food, or to eat too much food or to miss your activity program.
   - **Manage** yourself so that difficult times, such as holidays or vacations, don't steer you away from keeping your goals.
   - **Manage stress** in order to learn how to handle problems with emotional eating.
   - **Learn mind control** so that you can handle difficult and high-risk situations.
5) **Meet Regularly** with your support person or group.
6) **Practice for a Long Time** on getting these tasks to be a part of your lifestyle. The longer you work at it, the more you will get into auto-pilot. These personal skills become part of the way you live. Then, you succeed.

The first 3 recommendations from the experts are the basis of Dr. Ellis's 100/100 Plan. The Caltrac is a major breakthrough. For the very first time, you can monitor your efforts and see your results. With Caltrac, you take the guesswork out of your program. You have your own personal coach with you every step of the way.

Other behavior experts say that people who are successful in losing and keeping weight off *do not* rely on a complicated set of behavior self-management methods. They do 3 simple things all the time:

1) **Watch what they eat**.
2) **Exercise regularly**.

3) Weigh themselves. About this: how many times do you hear people say not to weigh yourself? Many weight loss "experts" recommend not weighing yourself at the top of their list. What fools! Weighing yourself is one of the most powerful regulators in the weight loss and weight control equation. Just remember, that your bodyweight will probably range within a 5-pound spread each day.

Folks, this is how to do it. Diets alone don't work. Move more, watch what you eat and count your calories (or learn portion control until what you eat in food volume allows you to maintain your weight where you want it), and weigh less. That's Dr. Ellis's 100/100 Plan.

Of all the experts' recommendations, **Self-Monitoring** is the key. It's the core of all behavior programs. People rank Self-Monitoring as the single most helpful tool. It's the one most often used. All 4 of the items above are Self-Monitoring methods. Self-Monitoring comprises 2 steps:

1) You must observe yourself
2) You must record what you observe.

With Dr. Ellis's 100/100 Plan, I encourage you to increase your activity. This is the most effective way to lose and to control your weight while improving your health. By increasing activity, you reduce your risk of getting killer and crippling diseases.

Self-Monitoring is the mainstay of your program. It leads to success and it's the most important behavior you can follow. Use your Caltrac as both a measurement tool and as a primary treatment strategy.

Self-recording of daily calorie burn lets you see how you're doing. It's a check on your behavior. Failure to burn what you need to burn leads to dissatisfaction.

Putting the Program Together & Dr. Ellis's 100/100 Plan

With this, you increase your motivation to burn more calories the next day and every day thereafter.

It is Self-Directed Behavior: changes you choose, changes you make. And they're based on scientific facts.

Caltrac can help you meet the goals you set. It doesn't let you off the hook. But it's not a nagging wife, husband, or friend. Caltrac gives you encouragement. It's you. You face yourself. And you answer only to yourself.

Chapter 16

Dr. Ellis's Version of the Low-Carbohydrate Diet

Even with the growing popularity of the low-carbohydrate diet, your choice to follow it will elicit negative comments from family, friends, and even doctors. Here's your defense: A low-carbohydrate diet used for weight loss has been proven to be:

1) Lower in fat than a diet of mixed foods,
2) Adequate in all important nutrients,
3) And lower in calories than a normal mixed diet *or* a low-fat diet. Also, rather than raising cholesterol and triglyceride levels, as is so often incorrectly claimed, this diet tends to lower cholesterol and significantly lowers triglycerides.

As bodyweight decreases, Metabolic Adaptations, aimed at preserving the status quo bodyweight, kick in, leading to the over-consumption of calories. ***At this point, it may become necessary for almost everyone to count calories in order to continue losing weight.*** Remember, the leaner you become, and the more you deplete your Fat Mass, the more likely it will be that you'll have to really pay attention to the number of calories you consume.

How Much Carbohydrate?

The number of carbohydrate grams that comprise a "true" low-carbohydrate diet varies, depending on your activity level and tastes, the amount of weight you want to lose (because of carbohydrates' affect on appetite and hunger), and the demands of your family during meals. (And it also depends on the author of the low-carbohydrate diet book, as we'll learn. Our task is to now

Dr. Ellis's Version of the Low-Carbohydrate Diet

clearly define the best number of carbohydrate grams to consume for best results and settle all of the confusion.)

The authors who have written on low-carbohydrate protocols rarely prescribe a diet comprising more than 60-85 grams of carbohydrate a day, and I agree with this, although, if you follow my complete program, you'll have more flexibility with how many grams you can consume each day. Sometimes active athletes can consume up to 125 grams a day although their performance would be better if they ate fewer. I know that consuming 13% of your calories as carbohydrate always works well. Just calculate your predicted calorie burn (or use the Caltrac to determine it) and do the math. For example, if you burn 2,500 calories a day, 13% of that is 325 calories. Divide that number by 4 to arrive at carbohydrate grams: 81 in this example.

Many writers argue that carbohydrate grams are the **critical factor in weight loss**.

They're wrong, of course.

These writers argue that you must find the "right" level of carbohydrates for weight loss, which may be as low as 10-45 grams a day. In my opinion 10-45 grams is too low for most people to tolerate; they'll never stick to consuming so few grams of carbohydrate. Based on your weight loss goals and dietary tastes, find a working point for yourself. I'll help you establish this number.

Remember, however, it's not the grams of carbohydrate that **directly** create weight loss; it's the effect of a carbohydrate-restricted diet which leads to a **reduced appetite, reduced hunger, and a subsequent reduced calorie intake. These, in turn, combine to lead to weight loss**.

Carbohydrate gram intake is not the critical factor, a fact, of course, that is in conflict with the belief held by some.

As a guide, if weight loss is your main goal, I suggest 60-80 grams a day *after* an adaptation period of at least several weeks. I'll describe, later in this chapter, the **exact steps** to follow during this adaptation period.

Therefore, if you're currently consuming 200 grams of carbohydrate a day, you might reduce this number to 150 grams a day during week 1, and then to 100-125 grams a day during week 2, and so on until you reach the level of 60-80 grams a day.

During the first 3-8 days, if you drop your carbohydrate grams to 5-20 grams recommended, for example, by using Atkins' plan, you may experience many side-effects including nausea, dizziness, and tiredness because the digestive and metabolic capacity of your body is set for carbohydrates and not fat.

These problems occur because, at first, your body is unable to use the fat fuel coming from both the fat you're eating and from your body's fat cells as a source of energy. Enzymes process the fat to provide energy, and it takes a week or more for the enzymes to really turn-on and to produce optimum energy from the fat fuel sources. It takes at least 4-24 weeks for these fat-burning enzymes to reach maximum levels in the cells of your body.

OK, be prepared for another proclamation from the Nay Sayers: Ketosis. Now, as we've learned, most people, including most physicians, believe that ketosis is dangerous and unhealthy. They're wrong, of course, as it's only unhealthy for people who are uncontrolled diabetics. In a normal person, ketones are a perfectly safe fuel for muscles, organs, and the brain. In time,

Dr. Ellis's Version of the Low-Carbohydrate Diet

even if one becomes ketotic, his body increases its enzymes to process ketones, and his blood levels will decrease. Don't fear ketones.

What to Do After Reaching Your Weight Loss Goal

After you've achieved your bodyweight and body fat goals by following Dr. Ellis's 100/100 Plan, you can gradually increase your carbohydrate intake as long as you maintain calorie balance. Don't go over about 25% of total daily calories (about 100 grams for someone living on 1,600 calories a each day and 190 grams for someone burning 3,000 calories). Always avoid sugar because it not only makes you fat, but it's also unhealthy. But even if you do eat a bunch of carbohydrates for a day or two, or during a vacation or holiday break, as long as you maintain calorie balance, it won't upset the apple cart. Maintaining calorie balance is the critical step.

Be careful, because if you eat too much food or too many carbohydrates (or a combination of both), it's easy to turn-on the fat-making machinery, and you'll start loading on those fat pounds all over again. And because of fuel-partitioning, carbohydrates convert to fat and are stored as body fat, creating a condition of starvation within muscles, organs, and the brain and then these tissues send out hunger signals. These signals drive one to overeat and become fat and also to suffer swings in energy that result from insulin's actions and changes in blood glucose levels.

"Hitting-the-Wall" or Reaching a <u>Plateau</u> in Weight Loss Before Reaching Your Weight Loss Goals

In working with the Atkins' recommendations (or any low-carbohydrate program) over many years, I've learned that people "hit-the-wall" with their weight loss. Some may lose 5 or 10 or 20 or even 30 pounds, but bodyweight loss *does* stop, often at a point **considerably** before one reaches his goal weight.

One of the main weaknesses (beyond not recognizing the legitimacy and importance of the calorie theory) of the Atkins' plan is its over-emphasis on the appearance of ketones in the urine. This over-emphasis on ketone excretion sets the individual up to fail because he will, inevitably, cease to spill ketones into his urine. When this occurs, the ketone sticks no longer turn purple (even if they ever did in the first place). Since this occurs to **everybody** and there is no explanation that this is one of the characteristics of **long-term compliance** to a low-carbohydrate eating plans, people, naturally, **become confused**.

Atkins argues that one must be in ketosis to achieve weight loss. When ketones fail to appear in the urine, Atkins advocates further reductions in the intake of carbohydrate grams from 60-80 (or lower depending on what Phase the dieter is in) to 40 or to even less than 20 grams. Even with further reductions in carbohydrates, however, the individual who has followed the diet for more than a few weeks fails to turn the sticks purple because he's no longer excreting ketones in his urine!

Most important is the fact that he doesn't lose weight.

Enter: extreme frustration and confusion.

What Atkins' book doesn't tell you is that, as the body's cells begin to burn ketones as fuel (ketones become the number one source of energy), there are simply no ketones left to spill over into the urine. The individual's liver continues to manufacture ketones, but he doesn't know this because the ketones are burned up and, hence, aren't available to spill over into the urine.

Dr. Ellis's Version of the Low-Carbohydrate Diet

Another error that impedes weight loss is that **Calories Do Count**. We must always remember this first principle.

Because of Metabolic Adaptations, including decreases in metabolic rate and bodyweight, the individual requires an ever-decreasing number of calories to maintain the ever-decreasing bodyweight, if it occurs. The failure to institute calorie restriction (or increased calorie burning) prevents continued weight loss because the individual is, now, simply in calorie balance, and no more weight can be lost -- **no matter how low the carbohydrate** -- unless he either eats fewer calories or begins to burn more calories through increased physical activity or combines both methods.

Metabolic Adaptations become more powerful as the Fat Mass grows ever smaller.

Of course, this is a major shortcoming of almost all diets today. This nonsense that **Calories Do Not Count** is so pervasive that it serves as the framework of many of the popular low-fat **and** low-carbohydrate regimens.

Most people think that just fat makes you fat, not that eating **too much food** makes you fat. It's logical to think that fat makes you fat, but biochemically, it's just not true. What's true is that carbohydrates, not fat, contribute more to fat making than does fat (although there's a large group of scientists who believe the opposite).

Dropping to a very low intake of carbohydrate grams can also lead to extreme fatigue in the first week or two when following a low-carbohydrate diet because one simply doesn't have the metabolic machinery to process fat as the cell's source of fuel, as I've described. The enzymes that break down fat (from triglycerides to free fatty acids and then to ketones) are in short supply. It takes at least 2-3 weeks for these enzymes to increase and, I believe, 3-6 months until they reach maximum capacity.

There is a <u>Big</u> Missing Ingredient in the *Dietary Approach* to Weight Loss: for both Low-Fat <u>and</u> Low-Carbohydrate Dietary Protocols

The key missing ingredient in all these programs is that the emphasis **remains on diet** and **not on increasing calorie burn**.

All the low-carbohydrate plans are more successful than cutting calories or low-fat diets because it's easier to eat less when one reduces carbohydrates. But most people don't reach their goal weight or goal body silhouette without increasing physical activity.

In summary, low-carbohydrate plans are more effective than low-fat plans, **but they're not the complete answer**. The major contribution to weight control and muscle building depends on increased physical activity. **All the proponents of low-carbohydrate plans miss the point: Calories Do Count.**

The low-carbohydrate advocates criticize low-fat programs as doomed to fail, yet their own protocols ultimately fail too because **their emphasis is primarily on dietary changes, and not on physical activity.** And, most often, the dietary change that they recommend misses the main point: **the importance of calories as the primary factor to manipulate in losing bodyweight.**

Dr. Ellis's Version of the Low-Carbohydrate Diet

Why Follow the Ellis Version of the Low-Carbohydrate Diet?

As we've learned, weight loss and weight control are *firstly* a function of the Energy Balance Equation and its two parts, Calories In and Calories Out. We've also learned that overweight and over-fat arise primarily from performing too little physical activity and then, secondarily, they're a function of issues pertaining to diet. Further, we've learned that weight problems rarely have anything to do with metabolic defects and are, in fact, related to behavioral and environmental pressures that an individual can, if he chooses, control.

The primary focus, therefore, to an effective program to control bodyweight is to burn more calories each day and to integrate that approach to one that modifies slightly one's calorie intake. An important contributor in using this second step is a diet that uses **Biological** methods to help control appetite and hunger and for this purpose, then, a low-carbohydrate diet is an effective strategy.

Here's the order, listing the most important factor in weight loss and weight control first, followed by those that are less important: 1) the Energy Balance Equation rules supremely, and the Calories Out side is more important than the Calories In side. What's this mean? Burn more calories as the first step, 2) reduce calorie intake using a diet of any composition as a second step, and 3) use a diet composition that's low in carbohydrates to help control calorie intake as a third step. Please note the order and realize that the low-carbohydrate diet is down on the list a few notches in its order of importance in weight loss and weight control.

Why is this important? It's because by using the most important factors first in designing your plan, along with integrating other effective secondary and tertiary strategies with it, you'll have, in hand, a program that possesses maximum levels of flexibility and a high potential for success.

In this way, you can choose to emphasize some parts, or mix and match several parts, to individualize your program to meet your needs. You can even vary your emphasis on different parts throughout the year, say, concentrating more on exercise for six months and then on diet for the other six months. This is a very powerful and effective approach. It prevents the inevitable boredom.

We must de-emphasize the belief in the idea of an overarching importance of carbohydrates to weight control. By rejecting that idea, we're no longer imprisoned to follow the very restrictive, and daunting, versions of low-carbohydrate diets that dramatically reduce the number of carbohydrate grams that you must consume each day for the rest of your life to succeed at weight loss and weight control.

My plan, therefore, provides more flexibility than other low-carbohydrate diets, precisely for the reason that my plan recognizes the low-level contribution of diet composition to weight loss and weight control.

Let's look, for example, at the Atkins' plan. He states on page 221 of his book, "On this diet, your rate of weight loss is generally proportional to your exclusion of carbohydrates." And on page 216, "This book is primarily about diet, and quite frankly, my experience has been that diet matters more than any other single thing."

Atkins explains to us in his book that he has performed a good deal of scientific research concluding that weight loss is proportional to carbohydrate gram intake. But, to reiterate, weight loss isn't proportional to **carbohydrate restriction**, but is, in fact, related directly to **calorie restriction** or, more precisely, to a calorie

Dr. Ellis's Version of the Low-Carbohydrate Diet

imbalance. Further, weight loss is more strictly related to calorie burn than to calorie intake and, therefore, it's not primarily a function of diet, but of physical activity.

These true, and well-researched scientific facts, are thoroughly understood and known by scientists in 2002.

My version of the low-carbohydrate diet recognizes that there's a threshold of carbohydrate intake at which positive results accrue from using diet composition as one of **several** strategies for bodyweight loss and control. That threshold is when carbohydrates drop below 25% of one's total daily calorie intake. That's more liberal than the protocol advised by Atkins. For example, for one who burns 2,000 calories a day, he gets to eat 500 calories as carbohydrate: that's 125 grams. A 2,500 calorie burner gets to consume 156 grams of carbohydrate a day.

Would you receive better results eating 13% of your calories as carbohydrate? Probably. But, are you planning to enter a bodybuilding contest, or fitness test, or participate in athletic events any time soon? If not, then reducing carbohydrates to such low levels is unnecessary, unless you **need** to do it to help control your appetite and hunger.

Controlling appetite and hunger is the most important reason for following a low-carbohydrate diet. By finding out how many grams of carbohydrate you need to eat to control hunger will individualize the program for your needs. **That's the right way to use the diet composition tool.** With such a wide range of carbohydrate grams to choose from, and realizing that it's a game of time, eating more on one day and less on another day is another strategy that will prove effective.

This is a plan that is far less restrictive toward carbohydrate intake because it's based on true scientific facts and has its priorities straight.

It's your choice: no dietary freedom, stuck for the rest of your life failing at weight loss because you bought into the idea that carbohydrates, and not calories, control the weight control equation. We must allay the public's confusion as to what issue is at the apex of bodyweight regulation.

One of my solutions isn't a dramatic reduction in and consumption of a very low level of carbohydrates. Using my version provides flexibility and avoids the efforts to think about a Critical Carbohydrate Level.

How to Follow the Ellis Version of the Low-Carbohydrate Diet

I'm going to present now a specific strategy for you to follow, but I don't want to lock you into the idea that this is the only way to follow a low-carbohydrate diet. I'm not opposed to starting out the way Atkins recommends by immediately severely limiting carbohydrate intake. If that's what you want to do, then that's fine. I'm pointing out that it's not necessary to start out this way for success. And further, you'll suffer from all of the "symptoms" the critics dredge up if you severely restrict carbohydrates. But, if that's what you want to experiment with, be my guest. These symptoms will all pass and are, in no way, dangerous. So, again, my Plan provides an extraordinary amount of flexibility so that you can follow a variation that fulfills your needs.

Let's review how to use Dr. Ellis's System and its Low-Carbohydrate Eating Plan:

Dr. Ellis's Version of the Low-Carbohydrate Diet

Week 1	Step 1:	Review the contents of this book. Study the charts that list the carbohydrate grams for different foods.
	Step 2:	Learn which foods are essentially free of carbohydrates.
	Step 3:	Continue your regular diet for the first week and count how many grams of carbohydrate you eat each day, creating your baseline. Continue to review this book and imbed its ideas into your mind. View yourself in different situations (at work, at home, at parties). Think about what you can eat during these times.
	Step 4:	Keep telling yourself that this is **not** a **no** carbohydrate diet. Keep telling yourself that you can eat some of the foods you're used to. Most people's first reaction is that they can never again eat any foods containing carbohydrates. Not true. You are supposed to enjoy this eating plan. They ask, "What about... [such and such foods]?" You can eat carbohydrates -- just not as many.
Week 2	Step 5:	Begin your low-carbohydrate eating plan. Your goal, if you are trying

		to lose weight and you are physically inactive, is 60-80 grams a day. So for this week, cut to about 100-125 grams a day. Continue reviewing the book, and think about adding a mild walking program to your daily activities.
Week 3	**Step 6:**	Cut your grams down to 80-100 a day, and begin your walking plan. Continue reviewing the book, and start planning some complex meals that are low in carbohydrates. A thick beef stew with rich red-wine gravy is an example of such a meal. Use carrots and potatoes to flavor the broth; just don't eat too many.
Week 4	**Step 7:**	If weight loss and control is your goal, cut down to 60-80 grams. You should have lost some weight by now. Keep in mind that most of the weight that you lose (about 70%) in the first week or two is the result of water loss, so weight loss will be much faster in the first two weeks, but this weight loss is **not** fat. Now, in the 3rd and 4th weeks, weight loss will slow up. Keep weighing yourself everyday. You should be

Dr. Ellis's Version of the Low-Carbohydrate Diet

		walking now. This adds some muscle weight, so don't expect the numbers on the scale to drop very fast. Your waistline, however, should now be getting smaller.
	Step 8:	Think about adding some weight training to your plan. Go to a sporting goods store and look at the 110-pound barbell sets and a good flat bench. Review some of the basic books on strength building. Study my <u>Spectrum Training System</u> about weight training. Don't look at any of the complex gym sets now. Up to about ten exercises with a barbell will work wonders.
Week 5	Step 9:	Keep with 60-80 grams. Watch the scale. Its numbers often stay the same for weeks at a time even though you're losing fat. Don't get discouraged. These numbers will drop eventually unless you're eating too many calories and/or you're too inactive. And remember, bodyweight fluctuates by several pounds a day because of water, so don't get discouraged if one day you are 3 pounds heavier than the day before. You must

		look at weight loss *averages* over several days and weeks.
Week 6 and beyond	**Step 10:**	Now you're in for the long haul. The newness and excitement *ARE OVER*. It's everyday now -- every long day. But this is where the results come. Build your program into your new lifestyle. Continue the mind treatments. It's all in what you think. This is the time you'll be challenged. If weight loss has stopped and you haven't reached your goals, you should not eat less right now, but increase your physical activity. If you eat more carbohydrates at a party or during a holiday, you'll repay the water debt. You didn't gain fat, it's water. Just get back on the plan and you'll flush the water out in a couple of days. This is where many people crash, believing that they gained 3 pounds of fat overnight. This, combined with the slower rate of weight loss that occurs as you move more deeply into the program, are the two biggest reasons for giving up. Don't give in. If you don't lose weight for several weeks, then you are

Dr. Ellis's Version of the Low-Carbohydrate Diet

		probably at weight maintenance. Tweak the 100/100 Plan a little so that you burn some more calories, and maybe eat a bit less.

Even though I've devoted many chapters to the discussion of what types of food to eat, I want to reaffirm the more important part of the Energy Balance Equation: physical activity.

Carbohydrate Grams in Foods and a Sample One Week Menu

The following foods are virtually carbohydrate free and you can eat them as you wish, but only if you don't eat more calories than you need.

Carbohydrate Free Foods

Meat	Fish	Fowl
Ham	Sardines	Cornish Hen
Pork	Flounder	Turkey
Lamb	Sole	Duck
Veal	Trout	Goose
Bacon	Salmon	Chicken
Beef	Tuna	Quail
Venison	Herring	Pheasant
Cheeseburgers (no roll)	Bass	Chicken roll (no filler)
Corned Beef	Bluefish	Turkey Loaf
Dried Beef	Cod	Smoked Turkey
Hamburgers	Haddock	Turkey Wings
Pastrami	Halibut	

Dr. Gregory Ellis's Ultimate Diet Secrets Lite

Sausages	Mackerel	
All meats are OK	*All fish are OK*	*All fowl are OK*

Shellfish	**Eggs**	**Cheese**
Crabmeat	Fried	Mozzarella
Squid	Omelets	Cream cheese
Lobster	Scrambled	Cow and goat
Shrimp	Soft Boiled	Cottage cheese
Mussels	Hard Boiled	Cheddar
Oysters	Deviled	Swiss
Clams	Poached	Aged and fresh
All shellfish are OK	*All eggs are OK*	*Most cheese is OK except spreads with carbohydrates*

Vegetables

Tomato	Turnips	Dandelion greens
Onion	Avocado	Artichoke hearts
Cauliflower	Brussel Sprouts	Hearts of palm
String or Wax Beans	Snow Pea Pods	Leeks
Broccoli	Sauerkraut	Bamboo Shoots
Scallions	Eggplant	Bean Sprouts
Spinach	Kale	Water Chestnuts
Asparagus	Kohlrabi	Chard
Cabbage	Chard	Rhubarb
Zucchini	Pumpkin	Spaghetti Squash

Dr. Ellis's Version of the Low-Carbohydrate Diet

| Summer Squash | Collard greens | |

Salad Greens

Lettuce	Chicory	Fennel
Romaine	Sorrel	Peppers
Endive	Parsley	Celery
Escarole	Chives	Alfalfa Sprouts
Arugula	Cucumber	Mushrooms
Radicchio	Radishes	Olives

Salad herbs, such as dill, thyme, and basil, are allowed, along with garnishes such as bacon bits, grated cheese, hard-boiled egg, and sour cream. All spices are acceptable as long as there is no sugar included in the product.

Fats and oils are also OK to use on the program. Many are important to good health. Use sources of gamma-linolenic acid (GLA) and omega-3 oils. Monounsaturated olive oil is a good product. All vegetable oils are permitted (preferably cold pressed).

Butter is also permitted but not margarine. Recent scientific research has implicated margarine as a dangerous product, one which significantly increases your risk (rate) of getting heart disease -- it's a health risk! Mayonnaise is allowed as is the fat on meat and under chicken skin.

Beverages

Water	Spring water
Essence Flavored Seltzer	Club soda
Decaf. coffee and tea	Herb tea (no sugar)
Diet Soda	Clear broth and bouillon
Iced tea (no sugar)	Lemon and lime juice

Cream (heavy)	

Carbohydrate Content of Common Foods

The following is a list of the carbohydrate content in some common foods that people consume daily. (Note: The abbreviation **gr. CHO** equals **grams of carbohydrate**.)

Cereals

Food	Serving Size	gr. CHO
Biscuit	2 small sweet or 3 med. plain	15
Bread (all except starch reduced)	1 slice, 1 ounce	15
Breakfast cereal (varies with brand)	2 tablespoons	20
Bagel	3 inch diameter	30
Bun, plain	2 oz.	25
fruit	2 oz.	30
iced	2 oz.	40
Cake, plain	2 oz.	35
cream	2 oz.	35
rich fruit, iced	2 oz.	40
Corn flour	1 oz. raw	25
Macaroni	2 oz. uncooked, 6 oz. cooked	50
Rice	1 oz. uncooked, 4 oz. cooked	20
Roll, bread	1-2 oz.	30

Dr. Ellis's Version of the Low-Carbohydrate Diet

Spaghetti	2 oz. uncooked, 6 oz. cooked	50
Tapioca	1 oz. uncooked, 4 oz. cooked	20
Vermicelli	2 oz. uncooked, 6 oz. cooked	45

Fruits

Food	Serving Size	gr. CHO
Apple	medium, 4 oz.	10
Apricot	medium, 2 oz.	5
Apricot, dried	6 halves, 1 oz.	10
Avocado	½ medium	5
Banana	4 oz., 1 medium	25
Blackberries	1 cup	18
Blueberries	1 cup	22
Cherries	4 oz. (1 cup)	15
Currants, black or red	2 oz.	5
Dates, dried	6 medium, 1 oz.	20
Figs, dried	2 medium, 1 oz.	15
Grapes	10 grapes	10
Grapefruit	½ fruit	10
Lemon	1 large	9
Melon	6 oz.	10
Orange	6 oz., 1 medium	18
Peach	4 oz., 1 medium	10
Pear, dried	2 halves, 1 oz.	15
Pear	5 oz., 1 medium	20
Pineapple	1 cup	21
Plums	1 medium	8
Prunes	2 medium, 1 oz.	5
Raisins	1 oz.	20
Raspberries	1 cup	17
Strawberries	1 cup	12

Tinned fruit in syrup	4 oz.	25
Tinned fruit juices, unsweetened	5 oz.	15
Orange juice	8 oz.	26
Grapefruit juice	8 oz.	23
Apple juice	6 oz.	20
Grape juice	6 oz.	30
Pineapple juice	6 oz.	25

Vegetables
(count all green vegetables as 0)

Food	Serving Size	gr. CHO
Artichoke, Jerusalem	4 oz.	5
Beans (cooked)	1 cup	33
Beans (snap, cooked or raw)	1 cup	7
Carrot	3 oz. (1 stick)	7
Corn	1 cup	31
Lentils	1 oz. raw, 2 oz. cooked	15
Parsnips	4 oz.	10
Peas, green	4 oz.	10
Potato	3 oz. (1 medium)	20
Tomato	4 oz. (1 medium)	5
Tomato Juice	4 oz.	5
Turnip	3 oz.	5

Dairy & Nuts

Food	Serving Size	gr. CHO
Milk, whole	8 oz.	11

Dr. Ellis's Version of the Low-Carbohydrate Diet

Milk, skim or non-fat	8 oz.	13
Buttermilk	8 oz.	10
Cottage Cheese	4 oz.	4
Cream Cheese	1 oz.	1
Yogurt, plain	8 oz.	20
Yogurt, fruit	8 oz.	32-49
Ice Cream	4 oz. (½ cup)	16-20
Almonds	1 oz.	7
Cashews	1 oz.	9
Peanuts	1 oz.	6
Mixed	1 oz.	7

Sweets, Sugars, Jams, and Soda

Food	Serving Size	gr. CHO
Chocolate	2 oz.	25
Custard	4 oz. prepared	10
Honey	½ oz.	13
Jams	½ oz.	10
Jellies, sweet	4 oz.	20
Molasses	½ oz.	10
Milk Puddings	4 oz.	25
Sweets	1 oz.	20
Sugar	½ oz.	15
Syrup	½ oz.	13
Soda, regular sugared	8 oz.	26

Dr. Gregory Ellis's Ultimate Diet Secrets Lite

One Week's Sample Menu

Sunday		Monday	
Breakfast	**Afternoon snack**	**Breakfast**	**Afternoon snack**
Scrambled Eggs	Cheese or meat Coffee or tea	Bacon & tomato	Cheese or meat
One piece bread/toast		One piece bread/toast	Coffee or tea
Butter		Butter	
Tea or coffee		Tea or coffee	
Mid-Morning	**Dinner**	**Mid-Morning**	**Dinner**
Tea or coffee	Baked fish	Tea or coffee	Lamb chops
Cottage cheese	Salad Cheese	Peanut butter & cracker	Green vegetables
	Butter		1 med. potato
Lunch	Milk	**Lunch**	Butter
Tomato soup	Coffee or tea	Melon	Cream cheese
Baked ham		Grilled steak	Coffee or tea
Cauliflower		Green salad	
Salad		Cream	

Dr. Ellis's Version of the Low-Carbohydrate Diet

	Tuesday	Wednesday	
Breakfast	**Afternoon snack**	**Breakfast**	**Afternoon snack**
Poached eggs 1 piece toast	Cheese or meat Coffee or tea	Cheese egg omelet	Cheese or meat
Butter Tea or coffee		Bacon or sausage	Coffee or tea
		Tea or coffee	
Mid-Morning	**Dinner**	**Mid-Morning**	**Dinner**
Tea or coffee Cheese	Beef or veal Salad Spinach	Tea or coffee Cottage cheese	Beef/ vegetable stew
	Chocolate soufflé		Tomato/ onion salad
	Coffee or tea		Coffee or tea
Lunch		**Lunch**	
Vegetable soup Baked meat		Stuffed tomatoes	
Carrots		Cheese salad	
Green vegetables		1 cup milk	
	Tea or coffee		Tea or coffee

Dr. Gregory Ellis's Ultimate Diet Secrets Lite

Thursday		Friday	
Breakfast	**Afternoon snack**	**Breakfast**	**Afternoon snack**
Grilled ham Cream cheese	Cheese or meat Coffee or tea	Fried eggs Sausage or	Cheese or meat
Orange Tea or coffee		bacon Toast w/butter	Coffee or tea
		Tea or coffee	
Mid-Morning	**Dinner**	**Mid-Morning**	**Dinner**
Tea or coffee Cottage cheese	Roast turkey w/gravy	Tea or coffee Cottage cheese	Barbecue brisket
	Salad		Salad
	Potato		Cheese
Lunch	Butter	**Lunch**	Small potato
Sliced lamb Green vegetable	Coffee or tea	Egg or tuna salad	Coffee or tea
Salad Roll		Peas or green beans	
Butter		Tomatoes	

Dr. Ellis's Version of the Low-Carbohydrate Diet

	Saturday
Breakfast	**Afternoon snack**
Ham steak & eggs	Cheese or meat Coffee or tea
1 piece bread	
Butter	
Tea or coffee	
Mid-Morning	**Dinner**
Tea or coffee Cottage cheese	Wiener- schnitzel
	Salad
	Peppers in olive oil
Lunch	Coffee or tea
Chicken soup	
Cheeseburger	
Sautéed onions	
Salad	

Chapter 17

The Science Underlying Dr. Ellis's Weight Loss Plan

You've now arrived at a place where you thoroughly understand everything there is to know about weight loss and weight control. Up until now, you've been a pawn in the weight control misinformation game. But today, you're the proud possessor of information that few others are aware of, including those in the medical and scientific community.

In this chapter, I will summarize some of the key points that you've learned and show you how I've used contemporary scientific facts to design Dr. Ellis's 100/100 Plan, a Plan presented to you earlier. There's no other plan that's as all encompassing, as powerful, or as effective.

The public is completely unaware of the fact that we scientists know everything we need to know, right now, to design an effective program for bodyweight regulation. The sad fact, however, is that many diet gurus concoct and sell plans for weight control that aren't based on **all** of the knowledge that's been uncovered over the last hundred years. Misinformation abounds, leading to the proliferation of an endless buffet of weight control choices.

I'm the first person to **piece together every fact needed for success** in weight control. Here's why: when I'd come to an understanding of **how the body works**, I designed a bulletproof program whose every strategy arose from a knowledge of all of the facts about how the body regulates its weight.

So many programs arise from misinformation and a failure of the program developer to understand the basic

The Science Underlying Dr. Ellis's Weight Loss Plan

facts upon which bodyweight regulation is controlled. I've covered many examples, but let me refresh you so that you'll understand what I mean.

The complex issue of bodyweight regulation is simplified when one comes to an understanding of the Energy Balance Equation. Unfortunately, few people understand that the Equation is the **overarching** factor in the control of bodyweight. Remember my survey in which more than 70% of the people polled said that the amount of fat eaten in a day was a more important factor in bodyweight regulation than the number of calories eaten? They were, of course, wrong. Although an understanding of the **One and Only Law** that's at the apex of bodyweight regulation is simple to grasp, embracing it has been, nonetheless, a difficult challenge because most people simply ignore it; many, in fact, actually refute its "fact-ness." Many so-called weight control "experts" actually out-and-out deny the existence of this Law of Nature.

Yet, **simple** as it is to understand the fact-ness of the Energy Balance Equation, this issue becomes **far more complex** when one learns that many things influence the Equation, leading to variations which make it difficult to apply its tenets to bodyweight regulation. Using the Equation as the basis for bodyweight regulation becomes complicated because -- when changes occur in bodyweight from following a diet or exercise program -- some of the simplistic assumptions about the Equation must be modified so that we can continue to make effective use of this Law.

We must possess all the facts as to how the Equation varies so that we can make the program adjustments that are necessary in order to compensate for these variations' effects. It's not that the Law changes; it doesn't change: Calories still control, but the body simply responds differently as changes in bodyweight, eating patterns, and exercise habits occur. A calorie measured in the laboratory on a desktop is a very different beast once it enters the body. Many changes occur in the Energy Balance Equation as a result of an individual attempting to make changes in his bodyweight. We must come to understand how changes in bodyweight affect the Energy Balance Equation because, without this understanding, the "weight-losing" individual will inevitably make many misinformed choices and decisions about the steps he must follow to succeed.

Not knowing about, or misunderstanding these variations, leads to the tremendous amount of confusion that characterizes bodyweight regulation and to the appearance of the never-ending stream of opinions and ideas about controlling bodyweight. Yet, there's absolutely no need for all the opinions because bodyweight regulation is controlled by **One Factor**, and **One Factor Only:** calorie balance.

When this concept is finally and thoroughly understood, we can begin to arrange and order all the factors that affect the Energy Balance Equation. Then we can build effective strategies for regulating bodyweight instead of following the shotgun approach that characterizes those who don't, first, learn all the facts.

Since no one else has ever put it all together, as I have here, the door was wide open for the production of my books.

Predictability of Changes in Bodyweight and Its Functions

We've learned, in the preceding chapters, that the body responds to changes in its weight in a predictable way. Scientists have mapped-out most of these changes, and as a result, we have a very good idea of what happens when one attempts to change his bodyweight.

The Science Underlying Dr. Ellis's Weight Loss Plan

My understanding of these changes prepared me to develop an effective plan, a plan based on facts and not on mythology. Having come to an understanding of **everything** related to bodyweight regulation, I have been able to design effective strategies to override some of the expected changes that occur in the "weight-losing" body, those changes that make it difficult for one to meet his goals.

For example, the vast majority of weight loss and weight control programs emphasize dieting (food restriction) as the primary method. Further, the proponents of diet as the primary method of bodyweight control often choose the low-fat diet as their recommended diet composition choice. Significant problems, however, are implicit in these two methods of bodyweight regulation.

First, scientific studies have convincingly demonstrated the limitations of the **dietary method** as a primary therapy, and, second, studies have shown that a low-fat diet is a poor strategy for effective bodyweight regulation because it drives carbohydrates into fat storage. Most of the ingested carbohydrates are converted into saturated animal fat and then stored as body fat. This process stimulates increases in hunger and appetite, a **DEATHBLOW**.

The first mistake is the false belief that a primary emphasis on the **Calories In** (dieting) portion of the Energy Balance Equation is the best way to regulate bodyweight. This method, in fact, has a poor prognosis for success. It's well established that overweight and obesity arise primarily because people are too physically inactive. Our sedentary, modern lifestyle is the primary cause of the overweight condition, not factors related to eating.

Some writers, such as Dr. Robert Atkins, have argued that a metabolic defect is involved in the overweight condition. **Serious** scientists, however, have clearly demonstrated that metabolic defects aren't implicated in the large-scale obesity epidemic. False conclusions, such as many authors have drawn, prevent them from designing truly effective bodyweight regulation strategies. It's only from a thorough understanding of all the contemporary, currently available scientific knowledge, that effective strategies can be developed.

The primary focus, therefore, of any bodyweight regulation program must be upon the **Calories Out** portion of the Energy Balance Equation. Failure to emphasize **Calories Out** makes it very difficult for most people to achieve their goals in bodyweight regulation.

Now, if you're unable to take the time, or muster-up the energy, to perform regular physical activity, then you are most likely doomed in your weight loss and weight control efforts.

That's a fact, sad to say, that you can't avoid, much as you might like to.

I've provided you with all the specific information that you need to design your own physical activity regimen. Resistance training should account for at least 50% of the time you invest in physical activity so that you can optimize your body's shape.

Reaching the appropriate threshold of physical activity each day, besides burning calories and shaping your body, is also a powerful **Biological** method to help control appetite and hunger because activity at the appropriate threshold directly affects the **Calories In** portion of the Energy Balance Equation.

Isn't that neat: concentrating on what you **burn** also controls what you **eat**. Two for the price of one. That's powerful! Controlling appetite and hunger is the most important factor in controlling the **Calories In** part of the Equation. The most **in**effective mechanism to control **Calories In** is the reliance upon Willpower.

Diet composition, as we've learned, contributes to Biologically controlling Calories In. The worst diet composition for controlling appetite and hunger is the mixed, or "super-market" diet, which is the type consumed by most people today. Most find it easy to justify following this diet composition because they live by a rule of "everything in moderation." Personally, I'm not a supporter of this rule and find that it's often incompatible with one achieving his goals. I avoid doing most things in moderation.

The Ellis version of the low-carbohydrate diet, in contrast to Dr. Atkins' version, provides far more flexibility in carbohydrate intake because my version recognizes the fact that diet and diet composition play a less important role in bodyweight regulation than Atkins believes. As a result of this fact, you aren't subjected to severe carbohydrate restriction. In contrast to Atkins' claims that his diet is "luxurious" (which it isn't), my plan opens up the possibilities of a more richly varied diet while still emphasizing the exceptional benefits provided by carbohydrate restriction. My diet is "every-day livable"; the Atkins diet isn't.

The popular low-fat diet also fails to control **Calories In**. Both the low-fat diet and the super-market diet cause carbohydrate-to-fat conversions, leading to storage of the newly formed fat (from carbohydrate) as fat tissue. This storage of fuel leads to a scenario in which the organs and muscles are deprived of fuel. As a result, these tissues' need for fuel stimulates the feeding center in the brain, commanding it to drive appetite and hunger, a process which, inevitably, causes the individual to consume more food. Only a diet composition that's low in carbohydrate maintains fuel levels in the blood that are conducive to reducing appetite and hunger drives.

This idea, of course, is contrary to what most believe.

Increases in **physical activity** and also a **diet composition that's low in carbohydrate** provide powerful **Biological** methods to help one control his bodyweight without relying upon the "guaranteed-to-fail" use of **Willpower**.

Changes in Body Composition

We've also learned that, as one loses bodyweight, both Fat Mass and Lean Body Mass are **companions** in this weight loss. Most people assume, wrongly, that when they lose ten pounds, that the lost 10 pounds is all fat. This isn't true; it's **absolutely** not true.

This companionship of fat and muscle loss (actually Lean Body Mass loss, composed of organs and muscles) varies, of course, depending upon principles that are well understood. Stimulating a proportionately greater amount of fat loss and a lesser amount of Lean Body Mass loss requires a thorough understanding of the methods characteristic of this task's achievement. These are the key strategies of my Plan.

A body possessing more Fat Mass at the start of a weight loss program loses proportionately more fat than Lean Body Mass. As one's body Fat Mass decreases, however, Lean Body Mass begins to represent an ever-increasing proportion of bodyweight loss. One's position along this continuum of tissue loss demands the use of specific (required) strategies to overcome these predictable changes. These strategies enhance fat loss and reduce Lean Body Mass loss. These effects take on a greater importance as one becomes leaner. I have all these required strategies built into the fabric of my overall Plan.

You must also remember that when beginning a period of calorie restriction, regardless of diet composition, up to 70% of the weight that's lost in the first 2-3 weeks is water: **Following a low-carbohydrate diet accentuates the amount of bodyweight loss that's water.** This is the mechanism that's <u>exploited</u> by Atkins and the other low-carbohydrate advocates; it accounts for the often large losses in bodyweight that characterizes the first two weeks of these dietary protocols, if it works, which it often doesn't. To account for such losses, otherwise, is simply hype -- or worse.

We're constantly pummeled, year in and year out, with the same sales pitches praising the next in the never-ending generations of weight loss methods, each guaranteed to trigger the loss of 10 pounds in 10 days or, better yet, 30 pounds in 30 days -- and all the endless variations in between. The checkout lines at the super-market counters are bursting with magazines whose covers proclaim the same misinformation. The marketing of pills, bottles, and potions promise "Just take this little pill. Forget exercise and dieting, and you'll find yourself in the promised land of weight control success." It amazes me that people continue to be hoodwinked by all this patent nonsense and magical hype.

But, since you've never been taught the 100% weight loss and weight control equation, it's easy for the shills to get over on you. That's over and done with. You've got the Power now, Baby.

My purpose in writing this book is to present all the facts, once and for all, in one place, between a front and back cover, so that **those who want** to invest themselves in an effective program will have every piece of information required to help them achieve success.

Why the Focus on Diet, Alone, Doesn't Work

I've taught you that your metabolic rate can be measured in a laboratory, or it can be accurately predicted by the use of a mathematical formula. The notion that people possess either a "fast" or "slow" metabolism is a myth. Some people, of course, do burn more calories than others because of their larger body size and because they lead a more physically active lifestyle. **But, this is easily measured and predictable.**

Don't fall for the old line that people's metabolisms vary wildly. The Resting Metabolic Rate is predictable and is based on body size. The Physical Activity Level of one's daily calorie burn is also predictable by the use of readily available tables for calculating the calorie cost of different activities -- or by using the Caltrac.

And increases in muscle don't lead to increases in the calories the body burns at rest, another false belief held by lay people and professionals alike.

What's the First Response of the Body to Calorie Restriction?

The first response to calorie restriction is a suppression in Resting Metabolic Rate. This is instantaneous, and its strength depends upon the amount of calorie restriction: more severe restrictions in food intake lead to a greater suppression of Resting Metabolic Rate. As bodyweight drops, there's a further reduction in metabolism as a result of carrying around less bodyweight. One way around this loss of bodyweight from fat loss, of course, is to increase muscle tissue as a result of following a resistance-training program.

The Science Underlying Dr. Ellis's Weight Loss Plan

If one has a lot of fat to lose, and loses it, he will never be able to compensate, pound for pound, for this large loss of fat weight by an increase in muscle weight because there are genetic limitations to increasing muscle tissue. It's much easier to increase fat weight than to increase muscle weight. The incredible proclamations of gains in muscle tissue (Body for Life by Bill Phillips as an example) achieved from following various training regimens or dietary protocols are mostly false, although there are exceptions: *every now and then*, there's a genetically gifted individual who can increase his muscle tissue to an extraordinary degree.

But please keep in mind, it's very unusual for a person to make these kinds of gains in a short time -- or, even in a long time. Then, of course, there are the steroid-using muscle guys from the muscle magazines who serve as examples of the bloated, false promises for this or that product or training program that we're told cannot fail to transform any one of us into a Mr. Universe or Ms. America.

Present day marketing messages use the popular "Before" and "After" technique to **dupe** unwary consumers about the value of a product. Again, the pictured subject in a before and after pose is only one, **of many**, who tried the product or program. He succeeded where others failed. We, of course, don't hear about the failures.

Often, though, the person pictured in the ad is a fabrication, manufactured in a computer graphics program. Remember the caveat posted at the bottom of the TV screen: **Results are not typical, individual variations may occur**. And for the magic weight loss pill, the caveat says that **exercise and diet are not required for success**. What a scam. If the product or program worked, **truly worked**, anyone would succeed who followed it. That's what happens if you do what I say; for everyone.

In what other ways does the metabolic rate change? There's a reduction in metabolic rate that occurs strictly as a function of the degree of Fat Mass depletion. The more the Fat Mass becomes depleted, the greater the suppression of metabolic rate. Obese persons, therefore, following a weight loss program, experience less metabolic rate suppression than less fat persons who attempt to lose weight because of their higher amount of Fat Mass. The greater the Fat Mass, the less the suppression in metabolic rate. Those subjects who experience more Fat Mass depletion will experience a stronger suppression of metabolic rate. They must be prepared to compensate for these adaptations or they will experience weight regain.

In addition to the suppression of metabolic rate with decreases in body Fat Mass, a drive arises from the depleted fat tissue that stimulates the feeding centers in the brain to increase appetite and hunger.

Our bodies appear to have a "fat-stores memory" that maintains the suppression of metabolic rate after body fat reduction. The apparent "goal" of the body's efforts is to restore the reduced Fat Mass to the pre-weight loss level. These drives lead to what we call post-starvation obesity. The body wants to restore both its Lean Body Mass and its Fat Mass, although the drive to restore Fat Mass is much stronger than the drive to restore Lean Body Mass.

What's the result of this drive?

When "finishing" a diet or weight loss effort, people begin to eat more -- too much more. The over-all acceleration in the gain of Fat Mass is more rapid than the gain of Lean Body Mass. Metabolic rate remains suppressed throughout this period of increased food intake. Although the suppressed metabolic rate increases to some degree with increased food consumption, the brakes are not entirely released: The depleted Fat Mass applies the brakes to the metabolic rate as a function of the body's "perceived need" to restore its still-depleted Fat Mass. Hunger and appetite drives also remain turned on.

Understanding these physiological mechanisms is what led to the development of Dr. Ellis's 100/100 Plan, with its emphasis upon increasing physical activity in contrast to most weight loss programs that emphasize reducing calorie intake. And the calorie intake reduction that I recommend, as we've learned, should be small so as to avoid these disastrous effects on metabolic rates. The use of calorie-restricted diets, the primary method recommended by writers today, is counter productive in the management of obesity and overweight precisely because of the physiological mechanisms I've described.

It must also be remembered that **it's difficult to become very lean and to maintain that lean body with its low levels of body fat** precisely because of the body's self-protective mechanisms. The greater the Fat Mass depletion, the greater the stimulation of drives to increase hunger and appetite, all of which leads to hyperphagia (ravenous overeating) and to weight regain. These mechanisms operate in everyone, but become stronger and stronger the leaner one becomes.

Metabolic Control of Food Intake and How Diet Composition Drives It

I've described to you the idea of the Metabolic Control of Food Intake, a control mechanism whose function is based upon the availability of calories (energy) to the active tissues, the muscles and organs. It's now understood that **the availability of calories to the**

active tissues is what controls food intake. If we can make more calories available, therefore, to the active tissues, we can reduce appetite, hunger, and hyperphagia, thereby reducing calorie intake **Biologically** and not needing to invoke the use of ***Willpower.***

I've spent much time in this book explaining all the issues involved in diet composition, an area in which misinformation abounds. The opponents of the low-carbohydrate diet are just as misinformed as are the proponents of this diet type. This diet composition is effective primarily because it reduces appetite and hunger and it also causes higher losses of body fat and preserves Lean Body Mass; these differences, however, don't qualify as "miracles." The low-carbohydrate diet also overrides the physiological mechanisms I've described, above, those related to the attempts by the body to restore Fat Mass that's been depleted as a result of bodyweight loss.

It is, needless to say, important to possess and to use methods that override the body's natural attempt to restore its Fat Mass after having lost it. This attempt at restoration is, of course, driven by **Biological** controls that stimulate appetite and hunger. Increases in physical activity, combined with a low-carbohydrate diet (an effective version such as Dr. Ellis's, not Dr. Atkins'), contribute to an even more powerful **Biological** dynamic than the use of either one alone in overcoming the drive of appetite and hunger which arises from the depleted Fat Mass.

Without these two powerful techniques, it's virtually impossible to resist the **Biological** drives pushing for the restoration of the diet-depleted Fat Mass. All this is made even more complicated because this suppression in metabolism, above, remains in effect until **both** the Fat Mass and Lean Body Mass have been restored to pre-diet levels. Unfortunately, because of the accelerated increase in the body's attempt to restore its Fat Mass, it increases to a level significantly higher than it had been before the diet. The restoration of Lean Body Mass, a process that occurs more slowly than Fat Mass restoration, is finally able to turn-off both the suppression of metabolic rate and also the driving of appetite and hunger. But, unfortunately, by the time Lean Body Mass is fully restored, the Fat Mass has usually reached a level that's about 150% greater than it was before the diet!

Low-fat dietary methods, and even the super-market diet (high in fat and high in carbohydrate), stimulate the laying-down of more fat in fat tissue because of carbohydrate-to-fat conversion. In this scenario, then, hunger and appetite are driven by, 1) the depleted Fat Mass and also by, 2) the lack of available fuel for the active tissues. There's no way that you can design a worse, a more ineffective, program. And further, because most programs rely on the dietary control of bodyweight, the subject is denied the important benefits attended upon increases in physical activity because such activity is, at most, only a secondary consideration in the design of most programs.

In conclusion, a thorough understanding of the physiology and biochemistry of bodyweight gain and bodyweight loss has allowed me to develop **the most effective combination of strategic methods for bodyweight regulation**. There are many parts to my plan; this allows a subject to place more emphasis on one part and to reduce his reliance on another part, based on his individual preferences.

It's important, however, to keep in mind that I've provided you with a set of strategies that is **hierarchical in nature**. One strategy is more important than another, and it's essential to focus more attention on the most powerful strategies. For example, increases in physical activity are more powerful than relying on strategies that use only dietary methods for bodyweight control.

The Energy Balance Equation obeys the Laws of Nature, as does your body. As you make changes in your body, these changes affect the Energy Balance Equation, and you must constantly make adjustments in your program to account for the ever-changing Energy Balance Equation. A failure to account for the way that changes in bodyweight and diet composition and physical activity affect the Energy Balance Equation has led to profound confusion in the public's mind concerning bodyweight regulation.

This book represents the first time in history that anyone has put together all the pieces of the 100% weight control solution and organized them into a comprehensive and effective strategy for bodyweight regulation.

Metabolic Adaptations

The final point, the one that I believe is the most essential to a thorough understanding of bodyweight regulation, is that you must understand Metabolic Adaptations. I devoted a large section to the discussion of this important concept. A failure to understand the dynamics involved in Metabolic Adaptations guarantees failure in the quest to achieve bodyweight regulation.

Please spend some time reviewing that important section. Metabolic Adaptations become more powerful the leaner one becomes. As bodyweight decreases and Fat Mass is reduced, one has to make significant adjustments in both his calorie intake and calorie output. If maintenance of a new, lower bodyweight and lower level of body fat is the goal, one must understand that he can **never again** consume as much food as he once consumed or perform at the low levels of physical

The Science Underlying Dr. Ellis's Weight Loss Plan

activity that characterized the activity level at his earlier, and heavier, pre-loss bodyweight.

Conversely, if one eats whatever he chooses to eat, and avoids physical activity, he will continue to gain weight until he reaches a higher set-point beyond which weight gain eventually trails off and then ceases: the cost of sloth and gluttony having been, finally, accounted for.

This is the result of Metabolic Adaptations operating in a direction opposite to those that occur when a subject is losing weight. Losing weight leads to an increase in "metabolic efficiency" which spares calorie use, whereas an ever-increasing bodyweight leads to increases in "metabolic inefficiency," a wasting of calories, a small but significant contributor to stopping bodyweight increases. Increased bodyweight also leads to increases in energy expenditure as a response to the body's need to carry around the extra weight.

So, if you're "at-ease" with looking fat, and being fat, and if you like to eat, and hate to exercise, then this is your ticket: get fat. For a person to become significantly fat, he must really eat a lot and move very little. It's difficult to achieve a high level of body Fat Mass, but not impossible as we see every day on the streets.

My "Dr. Ellis's 100/100 Plan" is predicated upon the facts that I've taught you earlier; I'll now tell you exactly what happened to me when I applied these strategies in my own life. Although I had used many of them in my past attempts to control my own childhood obesity and then, later, to optimize my body, I'd never used them all at the same time. In fact, some of the strategies remained foggy to me until I began to bring the whole program together about three years ago. This is particularly true about my understanding of Metabolic Adaptations.

Chapter 18

How I Put All the Elements Together for the Winning Plan

Writing the Book

In the late fall of 1999, I made the landmark decision to write this book. I thought it was time to tell the true and complete weight loss and weight control story as no one else had ever told it before -- I was (and am) convinced that no one else has had the experience I've had that provided me with the necessary background for this story. I understood it all by that time and had become disgusted at the plethora of misinforming, useless weight control books and programs flooding the marketplace, confusing the public.

One of the key elements in my book plan was to prove that my weight control program worked. To do this, I would use myself as the guinea pig. The book wouldn't just be about losing weight, but it would be about optimizing muscle gain and fat loss too. Anyone can lose weight, but optimizing the process is another story.

As a result of my vast undertaking, plumbing the depths of training, diet, science, and all aspects of controlling one's body, I had gained invaluable insights into weight control and body shape optimization. I had identified that my failures in controlling weight and bodyweight when using existing plans were because of flaws or limitations in the programs available on weight control and body shaping. I now believed that I had come to possess a breadth of experience and academic training that would lead to effective solutions.

I would use all the methods that I'd learned during the preceding 43 plus years about sculpting my

How I Put All the Elements Together for the Winning Plan

physique. Part of my plan was the ridiculous decision (I learned later) to reduce my body fat to 5%, the body fat percent that I'd attained in the mid-1970's.

I planned to start losing weight (and fat) after the Christmas and New Year holidays of 1999, beginning my odyssey January 3, 2000. In developing my weight loss plan, I committed yet another blunder. Here was my weight loss plan: I would combine calorie cutting and a low-carbohydrate diet with exercise, lots of it. I decided to increase my walking to two 3-mile walks a day, one in the morning and one in the late afternoon, a doubling of my previous daily walking distance. I would continue with my two-hour weight training program, 3 days a week, eliminating one walk on the lifting days. And I'd slash my carbohydrate grams to below 60 a day and try to maintain about a 2,500-a-day calorie intake.

Here's the blunder: I made a straight line calculation that, if I reduced my calorie intake by X number of calories, I could reduce my body fat and bodyweight to X by a projected time in the future. This, of course, was (and is) the universally accepted method used by nutritional counselors in designing weight loss programs. Why would I do it any other way?

I projected that I would lose six pounds a month following my plan based on the calorie deficit I'd planned. But I had no idea at what bodyweight I'd attain a body fat of 5%. I'd been measured at 5% body fat in the mid-1970's at a bodyweight of 181 pounds. I knew that, now, I had more muscle on me than I had in those vegetarian years, so I hoped I'd reach 5% at a heavier bodyweight.

On January 3, 2000, I began. On that day I weighed 219 pounds. By the end of January, I reached my goal of a loss of six pounds, decreasing in bodyweight to 213 pounds. It was a breeze; the plan was working out just as it should.

February, however, brought an unexpected surprise: I lost only three pounds, having reached 210 pounds by the end of that month. The end of March brought more disappointment because I'd reached only 208 pounds, followed, at the end of April, by a loss down to 205 pounds.

Those Damned Metabolic Adaptations Strike

It was now time to make adjustments in the plan. What was happening still didn't make sense to me. I knew that my rate of weight loss was slowing, even though I was very rigorous in my eating and exercise habits, diligently following the plan I'd designed.

Obviously, I'd had this experience several times over the preceding decades, realizing that, as I lost weight, it became more difficult to continue losing. I didn't, however, really understand it and never, in the past, undertook any effort to unravel the mystery.

Needless to say, it wasn't something that anyone talked about either.

I remember talking with other trainers in the past about this phenomenon, but the calorie theory, as it stood, preached that if you eat fewer calories, you lose weight. I hadn't been ready, during those early experiences with this phenomenon, to dispute what the textbooks said. The conventional wisdom, then and now, is that each pound of fat contains 3,500 calories worth of energy (fuel), and if one simply reduces calorie intake, or burns more calories, he will lose weight in a very ***predictable*** manner.

This conventional "wisdom," obviously, was incorrect, but I didn't know how to make the adjustments necessary for its correction.

How I Put All the Elements Together for the Winning Plan

I figured that I would "up the ante," so I began to walk four miles, two times a day, and made further reductions in my calorie intake. This worked, and by the end of May, I had reached 200 pounds. June's weight losses accounted for only 2½ pounds, my bodyweight having reached 197½ pounds, even with the manifestly severe increase in calorie burning and decrease in calorie intake. This rate of weight loss was significantly less than what occurred by following a less strenuous regimen when starting to lose weight at 219 pounds. By the end of July, I recorded a weight of 193½ pounds for one day, but the 7-day average of my weight, during these days, was about 196.

Don't be fooled, however, that my first series of adjustments led to this loss. During my July vacation in 2000, I made a second adjustment and began walking three times a day, averaging 12 miles of walking for the day while making further cuts in my calorie intake.

In July, 2000, I hadn't yet started writing the book, but had been gathering and updating all my scientific research papers that I'd accumulated, since 1977, in preparation for keyboarding.

But more important, by this time at about 194 pounds, I'd stopped losing bodyweight, altogether, even with the significant calorie cutting and lots of exercise.

The fact that I was no longer losing bodyweight really began to eat at me. I had to find out what was going on. I began a major research project to uncover the reason(s) for my ever-slowing bodyweight losses.

It was now that I began to discover some of the most interesting scientific facts that I'd ever learned in all my 43 years in the bodyweight game. What I learned about were Metabolic Adaptations, a subject to which I devoted a large section in this book. Metabolic Adaptations comprise, in my view, one of the most important issues that anyone interested in losing weight (wherever they are on the body fat continuum -- from already lean [and wanting to lose more] or from very fat [and wanting not to be so fat anymore]) -- must understand.

Their importance is most critical to the **maintenance** of bodyweight losses. I've never read a popular book, magazine article, or scientific book that discusses this important topic. In fact, what one reads, or hears, all the time, is that if one follows "such and such" program that he can simply *increase* his metabolism, not have it *decrease* as it actually does, easily reaching his goal weight just like that. And they all preach this -- how easy it is.

This idea of easily increasing metabolism so that one can eat more and still lose weight is pervasive in the culture and in many weight loss programs. It's an abominable mistake.

I won't elaborate on the facts, here, about the true story of what happens to metabolism because you should now understand from reading the earlier section what was happening to me. If you don't understand the importance of Metabolic Adaptations, reread that section; it's absolutely critical to the success of any program whose goal is to lose fat and to maintain the fat loss.

The problem now was what to do about my body's reluctance to lose any more weight. I looked very good and had gotten my abdominal muscles back, but I knew I wasn't yet at 5% body fat because I had pictures of myself at that body fat percentage and it was clear that I was not as muscularly defined, now, as I had been then.

I was now beginning to wonder seriously, however, about my decision to reduce my body fat to 5%. As I began to understand the sacrifice and effort it would take

How I Put All the Elements Together for the Winning Plan

to go that low in body fat, I was questioning whether all that sacrifice and effort were worth it. I looked good; I asked myself, why go any lower?

Many years earlier I had come to a conclusion about training and dieting. I'd tried so many extreme methods of each and discovered that no extreme method was **sustainable**. I just couldn't keep it up. Therefore, when I returned, inevitably, to a more "normal" routine, I'd lose the hard-earned results that I'd achieved from following the insane diet or exercise program. That was the point: If I reached a certain level of improvement as a consequence of following an extreme method, I learned that, once I quit that extreme method, my body would return to what it had been before all the madness.

As a result of all this, I formulated an infallible rule: Don't do anything that you can't sustain. The two-hour weight training workout, the eight miles a day of walking, and the significantly calorie-reduced eating regimen were at the very edge of **sustainability**. I knew that I'd be unwilling to ramp-up any one of them, and, if the truth were told, I felt that simply to **sustain** the current level of commitment and effort might come to be too much.

My subsequent understanding of Metabolic Adaptations was, needless to say, quite an eye opener: I hadn't had the vaguest idea as to the magnitude of the body's survival response in the face of calorie deprivation and weight loss (particularly body fat loss). When I was younger, I could make myself do anything that I wanted to do; following extreme methods like fasting, or the 800-calorie Pep-Up drink, was duck soup. I could make myself do them. I didn't like it, but I did it.

But, now, at this age, I can't tolerate the use of such extreme methods, particularly when I look as good as I do. Ridding myself of all body fat was not necessary as my boyhood idols had fat on their bodies and the new, modern-day "ripped" look was a result of drugs and the passionate desire to win physique contests at all costs, paying whatever price was required. None of the "ripped" athletes remained ripped when the contest ended, rebounding to pre-contest fatness in a matter of days to weeks.

Attaining a level of no body fat was not necessary, and I'd come to realize that it wouldn't be possible to stay there: it wasn't **sustainable**. That's exactly why I never stayed at those very low levels of body fat very long because I'd used methods that were not **sustainable** and the results, as well, were not **sustainable**.

That's one of the major problems with weight control programs today: people use heroic measures to lose weight, measures that they cannot **sustain**. Then, they return to their old habits and regain their former weight, plus more.

No, one must do it more gradually, changing his lifestyle permanently if he is to succeed, defining, and redefining his goals as he goes. Further, he must understand Metabolic Adaptations and make the required adjustments to compensate for them. Therefore, weight loss goals must be proportionate to what one is willing to do to achieve those goals. If one can't endure the means to his goals, he must change his goals!

I Go Off the Edge Once Again

By the end of September, 2000, I had crept back up to between 196-198 pounds, partly because of the discouragement consequent to my newly-found deeper understanding of Metabolic Adaptations and of how difficult it was going to be to reach my goal. It was all finally sinking in: all my disparate experiences with

How I Put All the Elements Together for the Winning Plan

weight control over the years were congealing into a final deep "knowing" of the subject that I'd so long desired.

I enjoy drinking wine and consume it daily. I had no interest in discontinuing that and, therefore, concocted a scheme to increase my calorie burning so that I could outwit those damnable Metabolic Adaptations. This scheme, of course, was breaking my **sustainability** rule by once again "upping the ante."

I asked my wife if she could make me a vest so that I could carry weights while I walked. A former sporting goods store employee, Laurie knew that weighted vests were commercially available at a local sporting goods store. I purchased a vest that held up to 40 pounds in the form of cigar-shaped metal bars that one placed into properly sized pockets sewn into the vest.

In late October, 2000, I strapped on a 20-pound weighted vest and stepped off on my four-mile walk. The walk was exhausting, and my trapezius muscles, the ones running between the neck and the shoulders, ached and burned. I assume that this occurred because the weight pushed down on the shoulders, and as a protective mechanism, the trapezius muscle continually contracted in order to resist shoulder displacement, becoming exhausted in the effort. The erector muscles, along my spinal column, also became exhausted and so did the muscles in my thighs and hips, these in particular because they were doing the real work; my "traps" and erectors were simply supporting the additional weight.

But, incredibly, within days there was a major change that occurred in my body. My thighs and my buttock muscles grew rapidly. My ass was growing so much that it was getting in my way when I tried to arch back over it from a standing position.

Obviously, by this time, I had been training with weights for many years. One of my theories about training was to use as many different exercises as possible so as to attack as many muscles as possible in order to stimulate development in them because each had only a limited capacity for growth. So, I reasoned, one should exercise many different muscles and make them all grow; as a result of this, one could achieve the most muscular bodyweight, as well as the perception of muscular size. My Steve Reeves training program used many exercises, so I was comfortable with the number of muscles I was attacking.

But walking with the weighted vest was like nothing that I'd ever experienced: I was attacking muscles that were not involved in my weight training program, no matter how much I lifted. The stimulus provided by the weighted vest caused rapid growth throughout my whole body. Obviously, the reason I began to wear the weighted vest was simply to increase my calorie burning without having to invest more time in my walking regimen. The muscle growth, however, was totally unexpected.

I calculated that, for each 20 pounds I carried, I would increase my calorie burn by 1.6 calories a minute. Based on these calculations, I planned to gradually ratchet up the weight in the vest to the full 40 pounds. But after only two weeks, I went from 20 to 27 pounds and found that this increase wasn't too bad. So after only one day at 27 pounds, I said "What the hell" and loaded my vest to the full 40 pounds. That, however, proved to be a real shock to my system. But, I delighted in the fact that I was burning 3.2 calories more a minute, for an additional 192 calories per four-mile walk. This was an increase of almost 400 calories a day over the eight miles. I was going to kick the shit out of those damned Metabolic Adaptations!

How I Put All the Elements Together for the Winning Plan

With the arrival of the Christmas holidays, I began gradually to gain weight again, and at the end of the holiday season, the scale read 205 pounds, up from August's low value of 194.

Most of my research for the book had been completed by this time, and I'd accumulated extensive notes, fleshing-out an outline for the flow of the book. I planned to begin writing in January, 2001. I was still wrestling with my plan to drop to 5% body fat, wavering to give it up or to go on. I decided, here, to give it another try and get back on track with my plan to drop my body fat. This was a difficult decision, not as easy as it had been in December, 1999, before I knew what I was getting myself into. I was now realizing how difficult it would be to achieve this low percentage of body fat. In November, I'd purchased another 40 pound weight vest and laid out a plan to increase my weight carrying so that I'd be carrying 80 pounds by March 1, 2001, and burning, in the process, a staggering 6.4 more calories a minute than without the vests.

In December, I wore the 40-pound vest, plus an additional 10 pounds in the other vest, 50 pounds total. Late in December, I increased the new vest to 20 pounds so that I was now carrying 60 pounds over eight miles of walking each day. The additional calorie burning yield was 5 calories a minute, or 600 more a day. At the end of January, I increased my load to 70 pounds, planning to reach my goal of 80 pounds by March 1st.

These walks were no longer fun; they were grueling. Nothing hurt, in spite of what many people say about carrying weighted vests: my knees, my hips, my back were all fine except for the muscle fatigue. (In fact, I've told about 10 other people about the vests, and they all report excellent results from using them, with no injuries.) It was just the workload and the effort required from my muscles and breathing that was so tough.

The muscles burned and ached, and I dreaded climbing even the slightest incline. My breathing often reached maximum levels. But, nonetheless, I felt, that by the end of February, I had sufficiently adapted to the 70 pounds to warrant the increase of my carried weight to 80 pounds as of March 1st. It was my goal and, no matter what, it had to be accomplished (well, maybe not no matter what because I was constantly fighting the desire to do it and the reality of how difficult it was to succeed).

And, yes, I did reach my goal of carrying 80 pounds by March 1st. This was absolutely horrible, the hardest physical activity I've ever undertaken. I found that I could do a morning walk, an evening walk, the next morning's walk, and my weight workout the next afternoon, but I couldn't muster the energy to take the third day's morning walk with the 80 pounds. I was just too exhausted.

One morning, I had just climbed a steep grade, struggling to reach the peak of the hill. I was now counting my walking steps because it seemed to ease the pain. This hill required eighty-five steps. At the top, I was breathing so hard that I had to stop and bend over, placing my hands on my thighs right above my knees, panting like a dog on a hot summer day. At that moment, my wife and son drove up and found me stooped in this humbled position. They both had been convinced that I was killing myself with this routine, and my current appearance confirmed their opinions. My wife always made me tell her my walking route before leaving the house so that she could come and "rescue" me if it was necessary as she was absolutely convinced that I was at the least damaging myself.

How to Meet My Goals Was Becoming a Problem

There was another problem: even though I ramped up my exercise, severely restricted my carbohydrates, and

How I Put All the Elements Together for the Winning Plan

reduced my calorie intake -- I wasn't losing weight. All this had been a terrific batch of effort -- not to reach my goals! Surprisingly, into February and March, I began to notice that I was looking much more muscular, even though I was still 205 pounds. It was then that I realized that the weighted vest walking caused so much muscle growth that it was the acquisition of all this muscle that was one reason preventing me from losing bodyweight. By early March, I was more muscularly defined than I'd been in August, 2000, at 194 pounds. So the weighted vest walking had increased my muscle mass by at least 10 pounds.

This was, obviously, very surprising to me, but it all made sense from my many years of training and research into training and diet.

Carrying 80 pounds was, however, not **sustainable**. I started with that weight on March 1st and lasted until the end of April, 2001. I decided to save myself from the suffering and dumped the second 40-pound vest.

In May, 2001, one of my clients told me about a set of walking poles he had discovered, similar to the poles one uses in cross-country skiing. I investigated them. I knew from my work as an exercise physiologist that combined arm and leg work was the best fitness developer and calorie burner imaginable. I ordered a set of the poles, adding them to my walking routine.

My back muscles and shoulder muscles became exhausted during the first four-mile walk using the poles. I didn't have enough strength in those muscles to push as hard as one is supposed to push when using ski poles in cross-country skiing. Walking with the poles wiped me out so completely that I had to take a nap, something I never do, similar, in effect, to what occurred to me many years earlier when I took my first 3-mile walk.

The weakness and lack of strength in my back and shoulders changed over the next several weeks as these muscles became conditioned. The other plus was, of course, that now these little-used muscles also began to grow!

At the same time, I was meeting my goal of increased calorie burning because the poles have been shown to increase calorie burning in walking by between 25-50%. What was even more striking was that, even though I was burning more calories (and I should have felt the effort), my sense of effort actually decreased! What more could I ask for: increased calorie burning, increased muscle building, increased fat loss: all occurring at the same time and, seemingly at least, with less effort! It wasn't, of course, less effort, it just seemed like it because spreading the load over so much muscle tissue makes the workload seem easier.

So my body's appearance was changing dramatically as a result of all of my little devices. These were all unexpected pluses to my program that came about only because of my decision to write a book about **Ultimate Diet Secrets**. Before writing this book, I thought that I had all the answers. But both the writing and the preparing of myself for the photo session uncovered a myriad of unknown insights into the science of weight control.

I was still not losing weight, however, and hovered between 202-204, but I did look pretty good. The plan, of course, was to put my photograph on the cover of the book as proof positive of the excellent results one can achieve following my guidelines. It doesn't matter if one is an obese 300-pounder, or a bodybuilder or a fitness person wanting to optimize his body, my program will work for anyone.

How I Put All the Elements Together for the Winning Plan

Decreasing Calorie Needs From Metabolic Adaptations

And what about Metabolic Adaptations: How have they changed my calorie needs? I've calculated that I'm burning, according to standard mathematical nutritional calculations, about 4,500 calories a day. But, in reality, I'm probably eating between 3,000-3,500 calories a day and yet my bodyweight remains stable, neither increasing or decreasing. That doesn't seem to make any sense according to the Energy Balance Equation, does it?

Do you remember that I said for bodyweight to remain stable one must eat the same number of calories that he burns. But the standard calculations show that I'm burning 4,500 calories a day, yet I'm only eating 3,000-3,500 calories a day and my weight stays the same. It seems that I'm breaking the Laws of Nature. But actually, I'm not breaking them at all. What has happened is that my low body fat percent has led to Metabolic Adaptations causing my body to become more efficient. Metabolic Adaptations don't disavow the Energy Balance Equation, they only modify it.

Scientific research has yet to uncover information defining the many factors that are involved in increasing the body's metabolic "efficiency," an adaptation that allows the body to survive on fewer calories. There are many questions: Do we need less calories to perform the same amount of work when Metabolic Adaptations occur? Or are our bodies performing less work each day leading to less need for calories? It's probably a combination of both, as we've already learned. The Resting Metabolic Rates of weight-reduced individuals are less at their lower bodyweight then at their previous but higher bodyweight. There's a definite drop in calorie requirements because of bodyweight loss because there's not as much tissue to support to maintain its life. The bodyweight loss by itself, however, doesn't account for the **total** drop in Resting Metabolic Rate. Other factors are involved that we know little about.

In my own case, because of bodyweight and fat loss, the reality is that I must now consume 1,000-1,500 calories less a day than the mathematical formulas predict.

Obviously, increasing my muscle mass by 10 pounds did nothing to overcome the Metabolic Adaptations by turning me into a calorie and fat burning dynamo, as many modern-day "experts" would have one believe.

On September 3, 2001, I weighed 200 pounds, a decrease in bodyweight of 19 pounds since January 3, 2000. I've shown, previously, that for each pound of bodyweight that one loses, he must decrease his daily intake of food by some amount of calories per pound lost to avoid regaining the lost bodyweight. The amount of decrease in calorie intake looks like it ranges between 10-50 calories a pound with those still possessing a good amount of fat needing to reduce their calorie intake by the lower amount and leaner people having to decrease their intake by an amount from the higher end of the range. For example, in my case, using 20 calories for each pound lost, the calculation for the 19 pounds that I lost shows that my daily calorie needs at my lower bodyweight are 380 fewer calories a day to maintain the lower bodyweight (19 pounds times 20 calories for each pound lost).

But those calculations did not work out for me. In reality, I had to decrease my calorie intake by 1,000-1,500 calories a day to avoid regaining the lost bodyweight, an amount far greater than the amount calculated using the 20 calorie/pound figure.

As I've shown in the section on Metabolic Adaptations, there's a wide compensation range for calorie reduction in response to bodyweight loss and the

How I Put All the Elements Together for the Winning Plan

subsequent Metabolic Adaptations. Some of the determining factors include one's initial bodyweight and fat percent, his physical activity level, how much total bodyweight is lost, and how much fat tissue is lost.

The strongest driving force appears to be the amount of fat tissue loss. And the magnitude of Metabolic Adaptations also depends upon one's body fat percent: the lower the body fat percent, the stronger the Metabolic Adaptations. In other words, the less fat one has on his body, the more he must decrease his calorie intake for each pound lost to compensate for Metabolic Adaptations and to avoid weight regain. This is because the body defends its Fat Mass very strongly. The more fat one has on his body the less protective the body must be. But, as the Fat Mass becomes depleted, the body gets very stingy, doing all that it can to protect the remaining fat.

The most extreme Metabolic Adaptations recorded in the scientific literature were those seen in the conscientious objectors in the Minnesota study whose body fat was reduced to 5.3%. Their daily calorie needs decreased by 47 calories per pound of bodyweight lost. This contrasts the more "average" figures of between 10-20 calories per pound of bodyweight lost seen in other studies. The difference between the studies, of course, is related to the magnitude of the body fat losses which, in the Minnesota study, were about as far as the body can go. Body fat percentages of 5% are about as low as males can go.

The magnitude of the Metabolic Adaptations, therefore, is strongly related to the amount of body fat loss, as we've seen. The leaner one becomes, the more "energetically efficient" he becomes -- and more powerful Metabolic Adaptation occur.

If I used the figure of 47 calories per pound as the amount of calories that I had to reduce my daily food intake to maintain my lower bodyweight, then this calculates to burning 893 calories less per day. This figure is closer to reality as contrasted with the 380 calories a day calculated based on a 20-calorie per pound Metabolic Adaptation. My Metabolic Adaptation, therefore, has approached, or exceeded, the 47 calorie per pound value observed in the Minnesota study. This is, I believe, strictly a function of the fact that I was approaching 5% body fat.

Low levels of body fat send a strong signal to the brain to drive hunger and appetite. The purpose of these signals is to replenish the depleted tissues to their previous levels. These are strong in-born survival and adaptation mechanisms. The strength of the signals is dependent upon the absolute amount of fat tissue in the organism as reflected by the body fat percent.

My low-carbohydrate diet, however, provides fuel for the active tissues thereby reducing signals arising from these tissues that drive appetite and hunger.

On the other hand, a high-carbohydrate diet stimulates the process of carbohydrate-to-fat conversion which reduces fuel sources for the active tissues. These tissues, then, send powerful signals to the brain that stimulate hunger and appetite. I'm overriding the signals that would normally arise from the active tissues to drive hunger and appetite by eating a low-carbohydrate diet because this diet type provides fuel for the active tissues instead of sending fuel into fat storage. As a result of this diet type, I'm not hungry.

Metabolic Adaptations occur in response to bodyweight and body fat loss and do not appear to be affected by diet composition, although we're not completely sure of this (I'm sure, personally, that it has no effect).

How I Put All the Elements Together for the Winning Plan

In summary, standard calculations show that at my present activity level, I should be able to consume 4,500 calories a day. These calculations are only accurate over a narrow portion of the bodyweight/body fat continuum. If one deviates significantly upward or downward in bodyweight and body fat, than the standard calculations break apart. Atkins argues that the low-carbohydrate diet "wastes" calories and that people consuming a low-carbohydrate diet waste 600-900 calories a day. If, in my case, I used his formulation then I should be able to consume 5,100-5,400 calories a day (the calculated 4,500 plus the extra "wasted" calories as described by Atkins).

In reality, because of Metabolic Adaptations occurring with bodyweight/body fat loss, I actually had to reduce my calorie intake by about 50 calories per pound of bodyweight lost. At the new bodyweight and low body fat percent I could only consume 3,000-3,500 calories a day without regaining bodyweight and body fat.

And for the "add-muscle-and-turn-into-a-fat-and-calorie-burning-dynamo" crowd, forget it. I added more than 10 pounds of muscle, while losing that much in fat, and I was eating fewer calories after this happened, not more, as they would have one believe. The decreased Fat Mass is a strong factor in increasing metabolic efficiency, thereby reducing calorie needs.

Stimulating Thermogenesis Through Everyday Drugs

Thermogenesis, by definition, is the stimulation of heat production (calorie burning) and, of course, thermogenesis results because of an impact's having been made on the Energy Balance Equation.

Known as the "drugs of everyday life," caffeine, nicotine, and alcohol possess thermogenic properties. Smoking a pack of cigarettes a day raises the daily metabolic rate by 10%. The risks, however, of smoking far outweigh the benefit of its thermogenic effect. In contrast, however, caffeine is relatively safe in moderate amounts and is found in many beverages and in numerous over-the-counter pharmaceutical preparations. In commonly consumed doses, caffeine has been shown to increase Total Daily Energy Expenditure (TDEE) by 5% in obese people who have lost weight. Therefore, the effect of a moderate caffeine intake on daily energy expenditure is significant. The ingestion of caffeine may lead to a daily heat dissipation of about 100 calories a day.

A diet of severely restricted calorie intake may, however, reduce the positive effect of caffeine in stimulating thermogenesis.

Nicotine and caffeine act by interfering with the activity of the sympathetic nervous system. Caffeine is believed to directly increase intracellular cyclic AMP, which leads to chemical reactions involved in energy production.

It's only over the past 20 years, however, that the interest in thermogenic drugs has shifted toward a systematic search for ones that mimic the activity of the sympathetic nervous system. These drugs work by increasing the release of the heat-producing neurotransmitter, norepinephrine, a hormone involved in energy-balance regulation.

It's a diminished sympathetic nervous system activity after weight loss (which is an adaptive survival mechanism) that contributes to a diminished energy expenditure. Hence, it's the function of these everyday drugs to increase the activity of the sympathetic nervous system and increase the metabolic rate that drops in response to calorie restriction and/or weight loss.

How I Put All the Elements Together for the Winning Plan

In recent years, there's been a search for both old and novel sympathetic nervous system stimulators in an effort to increase thermogenesis. These include ephedrine, which stimulates norepinephrine release and has been shown to induce greater weight loss than placebo. Ephedrine is reasonably well tolerated, and its side effects, despite recent FDA outcries, are mild and transient. One of the false claims made by the FDA is that ephedrine is harmful to the cardiovascular system. In conflict with the FDA's viewpoint, the cardiovascular system's tolerance to ephedrine develops rapidly. But the body doesn't become tolerant to its thermogenic effects, and these effects continue to contribute to extra calorie burning.

Ephedrine's activity is increased by taking aspirin which acts synergistically with ephedrine to stimulate calorie burning. Methylxanthines (caffeine), found in coffee and cola beverages, also enhance the activity of ephedrine. The mechanisms involved include a sustained release of norepinephrine from the sympathetic nervous system and an elevation of cyclic AMP levels at the cellular level. Therefore, attempts by the body to counteract the effects of ephedrine-induced norepinephrine release are overcome by the concurrent use of agents such as ephedrine, caffeine, and aspirin. A combination of ephedrine and caffeine reduces appetite and increases thermogenesis (calorie burning), contributing to the reduction in bodyweight.

In a study of obese people consuming these products, it was found that weight losses were from 7-11 pounds more after 6 months of dieting than in subjects not consuming these products. The side effects of these mixtures were mild and transient: blood pressure and heart rate were unaffected during long-term treatment. In another study, a combination of ephedrine, aspirin, and caffeine, induced weight loss in obese subjects even without calorie restriction.

These substances have all been part of our traditional medicine for several decades and have proved to be safe drugs. The combination of ephedrine and caffeine is 20-29% more effective in weight loss than currently used pharmaceutical agents, leading to more fat loss and preservation of muscle tissue.

Ephedrine and caffeine cause weight loss by decreasing one's appetite, accounting for 75-80% of the weight loss. The stimulants also increase thermogenesis, accounting for 20-25% of the weight loss. Again, here, even with these substances, we see the importance of **appetite control** for weight loss. The combination of the low-carbohydrate diet, increased physical activity, and these "drugs" provides an extraordinarily powerful **Biological** control over appetite and hunger, largely reducing the need to exert **Willpower** controls over food intake.

During the first month of use, ephedrine may cause nervousness, agitation, restlessness, insomnia, and hand tremors. These effects tend to disappear with continued use. An effective source of ephedrine is ma huang, an herb used in Chinese medicine for more than 5,000 years. Its long history of use, with no published reports of toxicity when used as prescribed, indicate that ephedrine is safe despite the FDA's outcry. It's likely that their efforts to bounce ma huang out of the marketplace is to protect the lucrative pharmaceutical weight loss industry. They, of course, will never admit to that so they trump up the charges of danger in their role as the protector of the drug industry.

Green tea extract, rich in catechin polyphenols and caffeine, also increases calorie burning and fat burning in humans. Green tea extract increases Resting Metabolic Rate in humans by approximately 4%. In one study it averaged out that subjects burned an extra 78 calories a day. Studies indicate that the activity of green

How I Put All the Elements Together for the Winning Plan

tea extract in increasing metabolism is increased by combining it with ephedrine and caffeine, and green tea extract accomplishes its task without increasing the heart rate.

A combination of ephedrine and caffeine is a safe, inexpensive, and effective diet pill which increases fat loss while decreasing muscle loss. Various herbs can serve as a source of caffeine, and ma huang is a good source of ephedrine.

DIM (diindolylmethane) -- a natural phyto-nutrient (plant nutrient) found in cruciferous vegetables -- improves metabolism by adjusting the balance of testosterone and estrogen. This leads to a hormonal picture that is favorable to fat loss and muscle growth.

So, you can't say that I haven't given you something for nothing. These supplements, added to increased physical activity and a low-carbohydrate diet, are powerful features of my program.

All the Tools I Put Together

This book is the most comprehensive source of weight loss and weight control information ever published. I have left no stone unturned in my quest to understand weight loss and weight control and the methods required to optimize fat loss and muscle growth. Along the way, I've developed an extraordinary number of tools to assist in this process.

You can access all of these tools through my web site, www.ultimatedietsecrets.com. From there you are directed to my products web site at www.targetedbodysystems.com. The products include the Caltrac for measuring calorie burn, my tape measure body composition program, nutritional supplements, the weighted vest, and the walking poles.

These tools and the information I've provided in this book, **Ultimate Diet Secrets**, comprise the necessary parts of a successful weight loss and weight control program for anyone. Obese individuals, as well as already fit athletes, benefit from following my instructions. I wish it had been as easy for me to acquire this information as it has been for you through reading this book.

You'll never have to read anything else about weight control; everything that you could possibly want to know is contained within the pages of this book.

There are those who will criticize some of my teachings because they are at odds with the majority opinion. Many of my teachings, however, are broadly accepted because they are consistent with majority opinion. Everything that I've written in this book is authentic and authenticated. Criticism of it can have its origin only in the critic's misinformation. My conclusions throughout are agenda-free.

I wish you great success in achieving your bodyweight goals and hope that I have made a major contribution to dismantling the extraordinary amounts of misinformation and confusion that surround our attempts to achieve bodyweight control.

Focusing on "the" Major Issue Related to Bodyweight Regulation

I've taught that the first principle in bodyweight control is the Energy Balance Equation and that every method used to effect weight change must direct itself to this Equation. The first task then is to teach people about the validity of calorie balance. This is a formidable task.

Why so?

How I Put All the Elements Together for the Winning Plan

Because so many "experts," such as Dr. Atkins who has influenced tens of millions of people, say that calories don't control weight. And many people complain that counting calories didn't work for them when trying to effect a change in their bodyweight. Confusion reigns, but it's all unnecessary because the Law is **absolutely** valid and controls each and every one of us.

I often sit with clients who swear that they don't eat much food, but still fail to lose weight. This false belief, that one consumes less food than he actually does, has been uncovered because of the development of the doubly-labeled water technique for measuring human energy expenditure. I described this technique earlier in Chapters 2 and 3. And what is the most important finding from the use of this technique?

It's that people under-report their food intake and over-report their exercise activity.

As conscious as I was of this fact, its total import only recently imprinted itself in my consciousness. I've now come to believe that the failure to accurately report food (calorie) intake may be the single most important impediment to people's regulation of their bodyweight.

And, no one is talking about it. No one realizes it!

We have to come to grips with the validity of the Energy Balance Equation and understand that the failure to see it at work in our lives is a result of our failure to report accurately the amount of food we eat and exercise we do. Until we understand this, there's no solution possible to the "failure-to-lose-weight-problem." Additionally, these studies have rendered most of the nutritional studies carried out during the last one hundred years useless and false. The data arising from them possesses no value.

The first problem to be solved is the under-reporting of food intake. Studies conducted over the last fifteen years confirm the fact that people under-report their food intake by a whopping 20-50% and over-report their physical activity by 50%! This failure to accurately report is what has led many scientific investigators to believe that there is some sort of metabolic defect that contributes to obesity. Even trained dieticians, who collect dietary data from subjects, under-reported their own food intake by 20%.

Biases in reporting food intake occur more often with increased bodyweight, lower income, less education, and lower overall socioeconomic status. Importantly, studies uniformly report that all groups under-report by an average of 20-50%. Further, research found that people under-report eating specific food types, such as fat and sugar, the "bad" foods, and over-report consuming the "good," supposedly healthy foods, such as foods containing vitamin C, fiber, and fruits and vegetables. It's also possible that the reported national reduction in fat intake actually hasn't occurred and people have only said that they're eating less fat because it's the "right" and "healthy" thing to do, PC, or Politically Correct.

These doubly-labeled water studies have also demonstrated the importance of physical activity in the prevention of weight gain. To reiterate what I've preached throughout these pages, physical activity must lead to the burning of at least 2,500 calories a week over and above the basic energy needs to maintain a new, lower bodyweight.

A Solution to the Problem of Under-Reporting

Researchers are proposing a valuable method to help identify those who under-report and the magnitude of their problem of under-reporting. In my view, an analysis of whether one is under-reporting is the most important

How I Put All the Elements Together for the Winning Plan

first step that an individual must make if he is serious about the control of his bodyweight.

Because of our use of the doubly-labeled water method, we have been able to make predictions of an individual's Total Daily Energy Expenditure (TDEE). These numbers are reflected in the data compiled by the World Health Organization (WHO).

WHO Energy Requirements (TDEE) According to Occupation			
	Light	Moderate	Heavy
Males	1.55	1.78	2.10
Females	1.56	1.64	1.82

To use these numbers to determine who is under-reporting, and the magnitude of that under-reporting, researchers have proposed comparing one's reported food intake to the numbers in the table, above. The first step is to calculate one's RMR from the standard formula I've provided in Chapter 3 and then multiply it by the appropriate factor in the table. For example, if the predicted RMR is 1,500 calories a day and the activity factor is 1.55, then the TDEE is 2,325 calories a day. If the subject reports a daily calorie intake of 1,800 a day, we can then use the ratio of his estimated calorie intake (the 1,800 that he reported) and divide that by his estimated RMR that we calculated using the formula for predicting his RMR. In this way, we can determine under-reporting.

In the above example, 1,800/1,500 = 1.2. If the intake was accurately reported, the ratio would be 2,325/1,500 = 1.55. A physical activity level less than 0.35 is not very likely unless someone is extraordinarily inactive physically; ratios less than 1.35, invariably, indicate under-reporting. This ratio plan, however, works much better at identifying under-reporters if we have an idea about a person's actual Physical Activity Level (PAL). Using just the table, above, requires guessing about PAL, and that has obvious limitations.

Since it's impossible to measure Physical Activity Levels (PAL) by the use of doubly-labeled water, investigators are exploring alternatives. Measures of home, leisure, and occupational physical activity (PAL) assist in determining upper and lower numbers that reflect whether the individual is under-reporting calorie intake.

The perfect tool for this job is the Caltrac. The use of the Caltrac to determine PAL may be the most important development in the history of people trying to regulate their bodyweight because the most profound limitation in bodyweight regulation is people's failure to accurately report food (calorie) intake. Until there's a solution to this problem, the use of the sophisticated tools and methods that I've described in this book won't help people: If one deludes himself by under-reporting what he's eating by 20-50%, and over-reports how much he's moving by 50%, then he's beyond the help of all these sophisticated tools and methods.

Delusion is the most common problem I fight every day in counseling my clients.

Caltrac predicts your RMR. Just put in your weight, height, sex, and age and place it on a table or night stand for 24 hours; then read the display and write down the figure for your RMR. When I developed the Caltrac software in 1992, I increased the formula-predicted RMR by 10% to account for the Thermic Effect of Food. After you read your RMR in the display, multiply it by 10% and subtract that amount from the RMR to obtain an accurate prediction of your RMR.

How I Put All the Elements Together for the Winning Plan

Next, wear your Caltrac for at least several 24-hour periods and write down the daily calorie count totals. Caltrac provides two different displays to get the information that you need: first, is the display CALS USED, which includes the calories of Resting Metabolic Rate (RMR), Thermic Effect of Food (TEF), and Physical Activity Level (PAL), your total daily calorie burn. Second, it also provides another display, CALS USED/ACTM, for just Physical Activity Calories (PAL). People will find this number useful in determining exactly how much they move.

The Caltrac predicts RMR, adds a 10% fudge factor to that number in order to account for the Thermic Effect of Food (TEF), and then counts your Physical Activity Level calories (PAL). Take the number displayed as CALS USED (which is the Total Daily Energy Expenditure [TDEE]) and divide it by your predicted RMR to arrive at your personal ratio of the multiple of RMR that accounts for your TDEE (which is CALS USED). Compare that to the number of calories you've calculated that you are eating, divided by your RMR.

Caltrac TDEE (CALS USED) divided by RMR should match or be very close to the total number of calories that you determined that you are eating divided by your RMR. If there's a discrepancy between the two ratios, then you are under-reporting your food intake; nothing else is possible, and I don't care how anal and detailed you think you are. Some are deluding themselves, others are just making counting errors by not viewing portion sizes correctly, but in either case using the Caltrac is a good method to get to the source of the problem.

What a powerful tool and what a powerful technique, probably the best combination ever created. It's clear that one of the most important road-blocks to weight control has been cleared-away in the past decade: the major barrier to weight control success, under-reporting calorie intake. At last we have in our weight control armamentarium the perfect method to correct that reflex of our human nature: under-reporting what we eat. I recommend that anyone interested in weight control use this technique as a first step before making any attempt to lose bodyweight.

We have also solved the problem that, more than any other, has confused the public in this matter of weight control. There's no longer any need for confusion because, as I've repeatedly said, we know all that we need to know in order to solve this problem. A detailed plan is in your hands, and it's impossible for this plan to fail. Each person can meet his goals if he just does what the plan says to do.

Where Do I Go From Here?

I believe I've added all the muscle that I can add within the framework of a **sustainable** exercise program. Someday, when I decide to give up my daily wine calories, perhaps I'll replace them with more protein to see whether that makes a difference.

I also have reduced my body fat to as low a level as I can tolerate. Whether I allow myself to regain 10-20 pounds so that I can eat more food than I now eat as a "restrained" eater remains to be seen.

I'm also playing with the idea of increasing my weighted vest walking poundage. I believe that I pushed myself much too fast in trying to add 10 pounds a month. It was, of course, OK at the lower poundage, but once I got above 50 pounds it became the old matter of "too much, too soon." I'm thinking of granting my body a much slower adaptation period, adding one pound a month to my walking poundage. In this way I'll gradually increase my walking poundage thus permitting my body

How I Put All the Elements Together for the Winning Plan

to strengthen over a longer period of time, allowing a full year to accommodate myself to an additional 10 pounds.

I'm curious whether 80 pounds will come to seem as effortless as 40 seems now, if I allow 4-5 years for adaptation. I remember when 40 pounds kicked my ass, and now it doesn't faze me. I will, most assuredly, continue to experiment with my body. I've spent so many years understanding how it works that it would be a waste not to continue using that knowledge.

Oh, by the way, I did make it into the 5% body fat range right around the time I turned 55 in April of 2002 at a bodyweight of 194, 13 pounds more weight than I carried in the 1970's when I had attained the same body fat percent. But, nonetheless, it was hard and I know I'll never stay there because that's harder still. But, at least I showed that I know **how** to do it and that I could do it a little more sensibly than I did it when I was in my twenties.

Well, in less than 5 years I'll turn sixty. My Mom always told me to give up weight training because I'd never stick to it as I grew older and it was a waste of time. I proved her wrong, needless to say, because I'm more interested now than ever before in seeing what exercise and diet can do to stave off the aging process. Maybe my next contribution will be to gerontology. Hell, I already qualify to be a member of AARP.

Good luck with the program.

Index

Activity level. *See* Physical Activity Level
Adaptations, metabolic. *See* Metabolic Adaptations
Adipose tissue. *See* Fat Mass
Aerobic capacity, definition of, 204
Aerobic exercise
   advantages of, 220
   characteristics of, 204
   effects of, 202–203
Age
   metabolic changes with, 208
   in Resting Metabolic Rate calculation, 30
   weight changes with, 218
Air Force diet, calorie counting in, 175
"All Gain, No Pain" slogan, 236-237
America College of Sports Medicine roundtable on physical activity and obesity, 197–199
Anaerobic exercise, effects of, 202–203
Anorexia nervosa, Metabolic Adaptations in, 109
Appetite and hunger, control of, 46–47, 127–128, 165–171
   after diet completion, 286–287
   diet composition and, 165, 287–290
   drugs for, 309–313
   insulin effects on, 158–159
   in low-carbohydrate diets, 177–178, 259–260
   physical activity effects on, 205–208, 280–281
Athletes
   Body Mass Index of, 44, 123
   caloric intake of, 209
   dietary fine-tuning in, 161

Athletes *(Continued)*
   glycogen loading in, 70
   Lean Body Mass of, 227
   set-point of, 118
   Total Daily Energy Expenditure in, 36–37
Atkins diet, 72
   analysis of, 195
   attacks on, 174–175
   calorie counting not required in, 175–176
   carbohydrate content of, 252
   failure of, 131, 132, 188–190
   false concepts in, 116, 280, 281–284
   ketosis in, 254–255
   theory of, 258–259
Autobiographical information, 1-7, 50–62, 93, 298–309

Balance, energy. *See* Energy Balance Equation
Behavior modification, 243–244
Beverages, in Ellis diet, 267–268
Blood cholesterol levels, dietary effects on, 179–180, 184
BMI. *See* Body Mass Index
Body composition. *See also* Fat Mass; Lean Body Mass
   animal studies of, 64
   calculation of, 43–45
   vs. carbohydrate dietary content, 155–158
   components of, 73
   determination of, underwater weighing for, 61
   after diet, 287–290
   gender differences in, 221–222
   goals for, 208–209
   in high-fat/low-carbohydrate diet, 135–136
   in low-carbohydrate diet, 151–154

Index

Body composition *(Continued)*
  in low-fat diet, 151–154
  measurement of, 64
  vs. Metabolic Adaptations, 122–124
  metabolic defects and, 74
  vs. metabolic efficiency, 110–112, 114–116
  in obesity, 79–82
  in overfeeding, 119–120
  physical activity effects on, 218–220
  post-starvation, 120
  preferences for, 208–209
  regulation of, 73–76
  resistance training effects on, 220–225
  variability of, 73
  weight change effects on, 68, 73–80, 90–92
    in fasting, 90–92
    gain, 79–80
    Lean Body Mass, 84–87
    loss, 77–79, 82–92, 282–283
    water, 88–90, 283
Body Mass Index
  of athletes, 123
  calculation of, 43–45
  gender differences in, 123
  vs. Metabolic Adaptations, 122–124
Bodybuilding
  Lean Body Mass in, 221–222
  marketing of, 285
  Resting Metabolic Rate prediction in, 227
Bodyweight. *See* Weight
Butter, in Ellis diet, 267

Cafeteria diet. *See* Mixed (supermarket) diet
Caffeine, in thermogenesis stimulation, 309–313
Calorie(s)
  balance of. *See* Energy Balance Equation

Calorie(s) *(Continued)*
  "body" vs. calorimeter, 115, 122
  burning of, 309–313
    vs. calorie intake, 167–168, 205–208
    Caltrac measurement of, 192–194, 237, 247, 249, 318–319
    daily rate of, 209–211
    fat vs. muscle, 228–231
    maximum rate of, 228
    measurement of, 192–194
    myths about, 225–228
    in obese vs. lean persons of same weight, 228
    by organs, 226–227, 230
    in Physical Activity, 228
    requirements for, 209–212
    in resting muscle, 226–227
    above RMR. *See* Physical Activity Level
    for weight loss, 214–216
    for weight maintenance, 214–216
  in carbohydrates, 184
  counting or ignoring of
    in Atkins diet, 175-176
    importance of, 23–24, 42, 161–162, 176–177
  definition of, 24
  in fat, 184
  listing of, in titrimetry, 38–43
  maintenance, 81–82
  measurement of, 24–27. *See also* Calorimetry
  partitioning of, 92, 136, 165-168
  requirements for, 81–82
    calculation of, 38–43
    Lean Body Mass, 109–110
    Metabolic Adaptations and, 115, 305–309
    vs. weight, 81–82, 115–118
  restriction of
    body response to, 284–286
    substitution table for, 238–239

Calorie(s) *(Continued)*
  sparing of, in underfeeding, 107–112
  under-reporting of, 26–27, 42, 242, 315–320
Calories Do Count Principle, 13–14, 20–22, 255
Calorimetry, 18
  calorie measurement by, vs. "body calorie," 115, 122
  for food energy content, 25
Caltrac, for calorie burn measurement, 192–194, 237, 247, 249, 318–319
Carbohydrate(s)
  calories per gram, 184
  complex, in diet program, 67–69
  conversion of, to fat, 133–137, 166–167, 183–184
  in diet composition, 129. *See also* High-carbohydrate diets; Low-carbohydrate diets
  energy density of, 143–144
  in foods, 265–271
  insulin release by, 162
  in low-carbohydrate diet, 250–253
  metabolism of, 146–148
  food intake and, 168–171
Cardiovascular disease-diet relationship, 178–180, 184
Cereals, carbohydrate content of, 268–269
Cheese, in Ellis diet, 266
Cholesterol levels, dietary effects on, 179–180, 184
Complex carbohydrates, in diet program, 67–69
Conservation of Energy principle, 12
Coronary artery disease, 178–180, 184
Council of Foods and Nutrition, on low-carbohydrate diets, 174–175, 178–185

Dairy products, carbohydrate content of, 270–271
Davis, Adele, nutritional program of, 50–53
Diet(s). *See also specific diets, e.g.,* Atkins diet
  complex carbohydrates in, 67–69
  composition of. *See* Diet composition
  discontinuation of, post-diet obesity after, 82
  Eskimo, 190–191
  formulas for, 50–53, 56–57
  heart disease and, 178–180, 184
  high-protein, 84–85
  ketogenic. *See* Low-carbohydrate diets
  low-carbohydrate. *See* Low-carbohydrate diets
  low-fat. *See* Low-fat diets
  mixed (supermarket). *See* Mixed (supermarket) diet
  with physical activity, weight loss with, 196–199
  resistance training combined with, recommendations for, 224–225
  success of, myths about, 17–19
  Very Low Calorie, 63–64, 84–85
Diet composition, 128–130. *See also specific diets*
  appetite control and, 280–281
  current recommendations for, 138–139
  debate over, 138–139, 142–144
  energy-partitioning and, 165–168
  food intake control and, 287–290
  obesity and, 183–184, 280–281
Digestion, calorie consumption in, 33

Index

DIM (diindolylmethane), in thermogenesis stimulation, 313
Dizziness, in low-carbohydrate diets, 183

Eggs
  cholesterol and, 184
  in Ellis diet, 266
Ehret, Arnold, Mucousless Diet Healing System, 60
Ellis 100/100 plan, 234–249
  advantages of, 281
  behavior modification methods and, 243–244
  description of, 234–235
  efficacy of, 236–237
  Energy Balance Equation and, 207
  500/500 variation of, 240–241
  Metabolic Adaptations in, 237, 240
  science underlying, 276–291
    body composition changes, 282–284
    calorie restriction response, 284–286
    Energy Balance Equation. See Energy Balance Equation
    food intake control, 287–290
    Metabolic Adaptations, 290–291. See also Metabolic Adaptations
    metabolic rate prediction, 284
    weight change prediction, 278–282
  step by step approach to using, 237–242
  300/300 variation of, 241
  variations on, 241–242
  for weight loss maintenance, 244–249
Ellis low-carbohydrate diet, 250–275. See also Ellis 100/100 plan

Ellis low-carbohydrate diet (Continued)
  advantages of, 250, 257–260
  appetite control in, 259–260
  carbohydrate content of, 250–253
  carbohydrate-free foods in, 265–268
  eating plan for, 260–265
  flexibility of, 257–258
  Metabolic Adaptations in, 255
  one week's sample menu for, 272–275
  physical activity with, 256
  table of food carbohydrate content for, 268–271
  weight loss goal of, diet after, 253
  weight loss plateau in, 253–256
Endurance, high-fat diet for, 71
Energy
  density of, in food, 143–144
  partitioning of, 92, 136, 165–168
  use of, at cellular level, 131–132
Energy Balance Equation, 194–195, 257
  appetite control and, 127–128, 165
  behavior modification and, 243–244
  calorie burn measurement for, 192–194
  components of, 126
  description of, 19–20
  in Ellis 100/100 plan, 234–235
  Energy-In side of, 24, 46–48, 126
  Energy-Out side of, 24, 46–48, 126
  energy-partitioning effects on, 136
  factors affecting, 24, 106
  fuel source and, 159

Energy Balance Equation
(Continued)
high-fat/low-carbohydrate diet
and, 133
imbalance of, obesity in, 217
importance of, 74, 161–162,
232–234, 277–278, 290,
314–315
low-carbohydrate diets and,
145–146
low-fat diets and, 139–141
Metabolic Adaptations
relationship with, 96, 136
rebalancing of, 207
set-point theory and, 106
unbalancing of, 22
Energy expenditure, total daily.
See Total Daily Energy
Expenditure
Entropy, 12–13
Enzymes
in energy-partitioning, 92, 166
in fat metabolism, 252, 255–
256
in metabolism regulation, 66–
67, 121
Ephedrine, in thermogenesis
stimulation, 311–313
Eskimo Diet, 190–191
Evolution, of fat storage
mechanisms, 137
Exercise prescription, 202–204

Fasting, 59–61, 90–92
Fat, dietary. *See also* High-fat
diets; Low-fat diets
calories per gram, 184
in diet composition, 129
in Ellis diet, 267
energy density of, 143–144
as fuel, 70, 131–132, 148–149
in low-carbohydrate diet, 172–
174
metabolism of, 150, 168–171
saturated, 179–180, 184
unfavorable reputation of, 130

Fat Mass
biochemistry of, 162–164
burning of, physical activity
effects on, 218
caloric content of, 97
carbohydrate conversion to,
133–137, 183–184
vs. carbohydrate dietary
content, 151–154
changes in, in weight loss, 68
energy storage in, during
overfeeding, 102
fat biochemistry in, 146–147
"fat-stores memory" of, 286
increase of, 79–80
leveling off, 217
after starvation, 119–125
insulin effects on, 158–159
loss of
vs. carbohydrate dietary
content, 155–158
as goal, 65–66
vs. Lean Body Mass loss,
77–79, 82–87, 119–121,
282–283
Metabolic Adaptations and,
286–287, 307–308
vs. water loss, 88–89
in weight loss, 82–83
metabolism of, vs. muscle,
228–231
in obesity, 79–82
resistance training effects on,
222–223
set-point for, 104–106
shape of, physical activity
effects on, 218
storage of, before overeating,
171
variability of, 75–76
Fatigue
in low-carbohydrate diets, 182
in vegetarianism, 191
Fatty acids, free, biochemistry of,
147–148
Fish, in Ellis diet, 265–266
Fitness revolution, 50–53

Index

Food
  carbohydrate content of, 265–271
  carbohydrate-free, 265–268
  energy content of. See Calorie(s)
  energy density of, 143–144
  intake of
    vs. calorie burning, 106–112, 205–208
    control of, 165–171, 287–290. See also Appetite and hunger
    daily calories in, 210
    energy-partitioning and, 165–168
    metabolic influences on, 167–171
    physical activity effects on, 205–208
    vs. Resting Metabolic Rate, 107–109
  macronutrients in, 128
  metabolism of, 150
  micronutrients in, 128
  thermic effect of, 33, 97–98, 100, 101, 213
Formula diets, Pep-Up, 50–53, 56–57
Free fatty acids, biochemistry of, 147–148
Fruits, carbohydrate content of, 269–270

Gender
  body composition and, 123, 221–222
  in Body Mass Index calculation, 44
  caloric intake and, 209–211
  Resting Metabolic Rate and, 30
  Total Daily Energy Expenditure and, 37, 213–214, 317
Genetic defects, in metabolism, 74
Glucagon, action of, 148

Glycogen
  loading of, 70
  storage of, 162
Green tea extract, in thermogenesis stimulation, 312–313

Heart disease-diet relationship, Council on Foods and Nutrition on, 178–180, 184
Heat, formation of, stimulation of, 309–313
Height
  in Body Mass Index calculation, 44
  vs. Lean Body Mass, in obesity, 80
  in Resting Metabolic Rate calculation, 30–31
High-carbohydrate diets, 130–131
  enzymes in, 182
  fuels in, 149
  insulin release in, 159
  lipogenesis in, 133–137
  weight loss in, vs. low-carbohydrate diets, 154–158
High-carbohydrate/low-fat diets, effects of, 151–154
High-fat diets, in Eskimo population, 190–191
High-fat/low-carbohydrate diets, body composition in, 135–136
Hunger. See Appetite and hunger
Hyperphagia, after food restriction, 170–171

Inactive Activity Zone, in physical activity, 206–212
Information sources, 313
Insulin
  action of, 149–150, 158–161
  release of, 158–159
    factors affecting, 147–148
    in low-carbohydrate diets, 147–148, 162–163

Ketones and ketosis, 146–149
  in Atkins diet, 254–255
  as fuel, 252–254
  in low-carbohydrate diets, 180–181
  pathological vs. physiological, 180
Kidney function, low-carbohydrate diet effects on, 186–187

Lean Body Mass
  of athletes, 227
  caloric consumption by, 108–110
  vs. carbohydrate dietary content, 151–154
  changes in, in weight loss, 68
  after diet, 286–287
  increase of, 79–80
  in overfeeding, 102
  loss of, 84–86
    in calorie cutting, 218
    in decreased physical activity, 218–220
    vs. Fat Mass loss, 77–79, 82–87, 119–121, 282–283
    Metabolic Adaptations in, 108–109
    in Very Low Calorie Diet, 63–64
    vs. water loss, 88–89
  in weight loss, 32, 82–87
  maintenance of, in diet, 64–66
  in obesity, 79–82
  post-starvation, 119–121
  preservation of, in weight loss, 84–86
  resistance training effects on, 220–225
  vs. Resting Metabolic Rate, 28–29
  set-point for, 104–106
  variability of, 75
Lipogenesis, 133–137
Liquid diets, 41, 50–53, 56–57

Liver
  free fatty acid metabolism in, 147–148
  glycogen synthesis in, 162
  lipogenesis in, 133–134
Low-carbohydrate diets, 145–164. See also specific diets, e.g., Atkins diet
  advantages of, 234
  body composition changes in, 151–154
  criticism against, 172–187
    on appetite control, 177–178
    on calorie counting, 176–177
    claims, 175–176
    correcting errors and, 185–186
    by Council of Foods and Nutrition, 174–175, 178–185
    on diet composition, 183–184
    on dizziness, 183
    on egg yolks, 184
    on fatigue, 182
    first major attack, 174–175
    on heart disease and blood lipids, 178–180
    on hunger control, 177–178
    on ketosis, 180–181
    on kidney damage, 186–187
    overview of, 172–174
    on uric acid formation, 181–182
    on weight loss, 177–178
  definition of, 129
  efficacy of, 145
  Ellis version of. See Ellis low-carbohydrate diet
  in Eskimo population, 190–191
  fat biochemistry in, 162–164
  food intake control and, 287–290
  fuel in, 148–149

Index

Low-carbohydrate diets *(Continued)*
  vs. high-carbohydrate diets, 154–158
  history of, 145–146
  insulin release in, 147–148, 158–159, 162–163
  ketogenesis in, 146–149
  mechanisms of, 131–132
  mineral intake in, 173
  minimum carbohydrate content of, 160–162
  unrestricted calorie intake in, 175–177
  vitamin intake in, 173
  weight gain after, 158
  weight loss in, vs. high-carbohydrate diets, 154–158
Low-fat diets, 138–143
  body composition in, 151–154
  debate over, 138–139, 142–144
  definition of, 129
  energy density of, 143–144
  failure of, 139–141, 278–282
  popularity of, 138, 142–143
Low-fat/high-carbohydrate diets, fat storage in, 170
Luxuskonsumption, in overfeeding, 103

Ma huang, in thermogenesis stimulation, 312
Mayer hypothesis, of food intake vs. calorie burning, 206–208, 212–214
Meat
  avoidance of (vegetarianism), 57–59, 130–131, 191
  carbohydrate-free nature of, 265–266
  as Eskimo diet, 190–191
  total diet of, 172–173
Menus, for Ellis diet, 272–275

Metabolic Adaptations, 15, 94–125
  adjustments for, in weight loss program, 110, 113–119
  in anorexia nervosa, 109
  vs. Body Mass Index, 122–124
  calorie needs and, 305–309
  definition of, 95
  discovery of, 294–295
  in Ellis 100/100 plan, 236, 237, 240
  in Ellis low-carbohydrate diet, 255
  Energy Balance Equation and, 96, 136
  Fat Mass loss and, 307–308
  vs. food intake, 106–112
  importance of, 95–96, 290–291
  vs. Lean Body Mass, 108–109
  in lean individuals, 96
  luxuskonsumption mechanism and, 103
  metabolic efficiency in, 90–91, 114–115
  in overfeeding, 102–103
  persistence of, 112
  Physical Activity Level and, 100–101, 107, 115
  in post-starvation obesity, 119–121
  Resting Metabolic Rate changes in, 100–101, 107–109, 115
  set-point theory and, 104–106, 111–112, 118–119
  survival advantage of, 118
  Total Daily Energy Expenditure and, 100–101, 103–104, 107, 115
  in weight loss, 113–119, 294–298
Metabolic rate
  determination of, 27–32
  resting. *See* Resting Metabolic Rate

Metabolic rate *(Continued)*
   types of, 27–28
Metabolism
   defects and differences in, 74
   myths about, 26, 225–231, 279–280, 284
   efficiency of, 99
   vs. body composition, 114–116
   in weight loss, 90–91, 110–112, 114–115
   in food intake control, 165–171
   regulation of, 66–67
Micronutrients, 128
Minerals, in low-carbohydrate diet, 173
Mixed (supermarket) diet
   definition of, 129
   fat metabolism in, 170
   fat storage in, 169
   obesity due to, 169, 280–281
Mucousless Diet Healing System, 60
Muscle
   building of (bodybuilding), 221–222, 227, 285
   calorie burning in, 226–227, 229–231
   maintenance of, in diet, 64–66
   metabolism of, vs. fat, 228–231
   resting, calorie burning in, 226–227
   volume of, genetic limitations of, 284–285
Myths
   about body composition changes, 282–284
   about diet program success, 17–19
   about exercise effects on appetite, 205
   about exercise effects on metabolic rate, 225–228
   about metabolism defects, 279–280, 284

Myths *(Continued)*
   about metabolism differences, 26, 228–231
   about weight loss diets, 279–280

Newtonian Laws, 11–16
Nicotine, in thermogenesis stimulation, 309–310
Non-resting energy expenditure. *See* Physical Activity Level
Normal Activity Zone, food intake in, 206–207

Obesity
   body composition in, 79–82
   calorie needs in, 81
   causes of, 48–49, 212–213, 216–217
   childhood, 4–7
   diet composition and, 183–184
   energy-partitioning and, 167
   heat dissipation in, 114
   metabolic inefficiency in, 110, 114
   post-starvation, 81–82, 119–125, 170–171
   sedentary lifestyle and, 206–208
   set-point and, 111, 217
   thermogenesis stimulation drugs for, 311
Occupation, vs. Total Daily Energy Expenditure, 36–37, 317
Oils, in Ellis diet, 267
Organs, calorie burning of, 226–227, 230
Overfeeding
   body composition in, 119–121
   effects of, 102–104
   after food restriction, 170–171

Pennington theory of weight control, 147–148
Pep-Up formula diet, 50–53, 56–57

Index

Physical activity. *See also* Physical Activity Level; Resistance/weight training
appetite impact of, 205–208
attitudes toward, 212, 233
body composition changes with, 218–220
calorie burning in, 209–212, 228
measurement with Caltrac, 192–194, 237, 247, 249, 318–319
with diet, weight loss with, 196–199, 278–282
duration of, in exercise prescription, 202–203
exercise prescription for, 202–204
in Fat Mass reduction, 197–198
frequency of, in exercise prescription, 202–203
health-related vs. performance-related, 204–205
importance of, 196–197, 256
Inactive Activity Zone in, 206–212
increase of
with Ellis low-carbohydrate diet, 256
for weight maintenance, 235–248
intensity of, in exercise prescription, 202–203
Mayer hypothesis of, 206–208, 212–214
with no diet change, weight loss in, 199–200
Normal Activity Zone in, 206–207
vs. obesity development, 216–217
recommended amount of, 214–216
time requirements for, 201–202, 212, 215
types of, 202–204, 220–221

Physical Activity *(Continued)*
weight effects of, 205–208
in weight loss, 197–198
Physical Activity Level
average, 239
vs. Body Mass Index, 214–216
calculation of, 213, 318
for Ellis 100/100 plan, 237
vs. Fat Mass, 214–216
increased, changes from, 218–220
low, in overweight development, 199–200
manipulation of, 46
Metabolic Adaptations and, 100–101, 107, 115
minimum, 208–209, 214–216
threshold of
for weight loss, 239
for weight maintenance, 216
too-low, weight gain in, 74
vs. Total Daily Energy Expenditure, 36–37, 215
Total Daily Energy Expenditure/Resting Metabolic Rate index for, 34–35
Physical culture movement, 50–53
Poles, walking, 303
Post-starvation obesity, 81–82, 119–121, 170–171
Protein, in diet composition, 129

Relapse prevention, in weight loss maintenance, 245
Resistance/weight training
benefits of, 221
body composition changes in, 220–225
diet combined with, recommendations for, 224–225
effects of, 202–203
for muscle maintenance, 64

331

Resting Metabolic Rate
  in active vs. non-active persons, 227–228
  average, 239
  in bodybuilding, prediction of, 227
  calculation of, 30–32, 237, 317
  calorie burning beyond, 216
  calorie restriction effects on, 284
  Caltrac prediction of, 318–319
  changes in, 31, 46
    in Metabolic Adaptations, 100–101, 107–109, 115
  decrease of
    phases of, 108
    in Very Low Calorie Diet, 63–64, 84
  definition of, 28
  factors affecting, 28–29
  vs. food intake, 107–109
  green tea extract effects on, 312
  vs. Lean Body Mass, 28–29
  measurement of, 29
  in obese vs. lean persons of same weight, 228
  in Physical Activity Level determination, 34–35, 213–214
  vs. Total Daily Energy Expenditure, 28, 100
  in Total Daily Energy Expenditure calculation, 36–37
  vs. weight, 28–29
RMR. *See* Resting Metabolic Rate

Salad greens, carbohydrate-free, 267
Sedentary life style
  food intake in, 206–208
  Total Daily Energy Expenditure in, 36
Self-monitoring, in weight loss program, 248–249
Semi-starvation
  Metabolic Adaptations to, 113–114
  water loss in, 88–89
Set-point theory, of weight, 104–106, 111–112, 115–119, 122
  in obesity, 111, 217
Smoking, in thermogenesis stimulation, 309–310
Social situations, relapse related to, 246
Social support, for weight loss maintenance, 245
Somers, Suzanne, diet of, 107, 176
Specific Dynamic Action, 33
Starvation. *See also* Fasting
  of active tissues, 168–171
  insulin release in, 147–148
  obesity after, 81–82, 119–125, 170–171
Stefansson, Vilhajalmur, on Eskimo Diet, 190–191
Stillman diet, calorie counting in, 175
Strength training. *See* Resistance/weight training
Supermarket diet. *See* Mixed (supermarket) diet
Sweets, carbohydrate content of, 271
Sympathetic nervous stimulation, for thermogenesis, 310–311

Taller diet, calorie counting in, 175
TDEE. *See* Total Daily Energy Expenditure
Thermic Effect of Food, 33, 97–98, 100, 101, 213
Thermodynamics, laws of, 11–16
Thermogenesis, stimulation of, 309–313
Titrimetry, 38–43

Index

Total Daily Energy Expenditure
vs. activity level, 36–37, 215
average, 239
caffeine effects on, 310
calculation of
accurate, 38–43
for Ellis 100/100 plan, 237
quick estimate, 34–36
Caltrac prediction of, 319
components of, 27–28, 33, 100–101, 213. *See also specific components*
determination of, 38–43
vs. gender, 213–214, 317
maximum, 36–37
Metabolic Adaptations and, 100–101, 107, 115
minimum, 36, 214–216
in obesity, 80
vs. occupation, 317
in Physical Activity Level determination, 213–214
range of, 36–37
reduction of, in underfeeding, 103
vs. Resting Metabolic Rate, 100–101
Thermic Effect of Food in, 33
titrimetry based on, 38–43
Total Daily Energy Expenditure/Resting Metabolic Rate index, 34–35, 213–214
Triglycerides
blood levels of, in low-carbohydrate diets, 179–180
burning of, 149–150
fat storage as, 146–147

Underfeeding. *See also* Starvation
calorie sparing in, 106–112, 107–112
in fasting, 59–61, 90–92
in semi-starvation, 88–89, 113–114

Underfeeding *(Continued)*
Total Daily Energy Expenditure reduction in, 103
Underwater weighing, for body composition determination, 61
Uric acid formation, in low-carbohydrate diets, 181–182

Vegetables
carbohydrate content of, 270
carbohydrate-free, 266–267
Vegetarianism, 56, 58–59, 130–131, 191
Very Low Calorie Diet, 63–64, 84–85
Vest, weighted, for walking, 299–304, 320–321
Vitamin(s), in low-carbohydrate diet, 173

Walking, with weighted vest, 299–304, 320–321
Water, loss of
vs. carbohydrate dietary content, 156–158
in low-carbohydrate diets, 177
in weight loss, 88–90, 283
Web site, 313
Weight. *See also* Weight gain; Weight loss
in Body Mass Index calculation, 44
changes of, prediction of, 278–282
measurement of, importance of, 247
vs. Resting Metabolic Rate, 28–29
in Resting Metabolic Rate calculation, 30–31
set-point theory of, 111–112, 118–119
wide fluctuations of, 53–61, 93
Weight gain
body composition changes with, 79–82

333

Weight gain *(Continued)*
  after diet
    diet composition and, 287–290
    low-carbohydrate, 158
  in overfeeding, 102–103
Weight loss
  body composition changes with, 77–79, 82–92, 282–283
  vs. carbohydrate dietary content, 151–158
  difficulty of, 107, 112, 117–119, 124, 125
  in fasting, 90–92
  fat metabolism after, 169–170
  goals of, diet after, 253
  Lean Body Mass loss in, 32
  in low-carbohydrate diets, 177–178
  maintenance of, 244–249
    Metabolic Adaptations and, 294–298
    problems with, 246
    steps for, 246–247
  Metabolic Adaptations in. *See* Metabolic Adaptations
  physical activity vs. diet roles in, 196–199, 278–282
  symptoms after, 60, 105
  water loss in, 88–90, 283
Weight training. *See* Resistance/weight training
Willpower, in appetite control, 46–47
  difficulty of, 116–117, 127–128, 165, 281
World Health Organization
  Total Daily Energy Expenditure requirements of, 36
  Total Daily Energy Expenditure/Resting Metabolic Rate index of, 34-35

Ultimate Diet Secrets.com
Dr. Gregory Ellis's 100% Weight Loss and Weight Control Solution

Quick Order Form

- **Fax Orders:** 610-558-1287. Send this form.
- **Telephone Orders:** Call 800-337-7041 (orders only). Have your credit card information ready.
- **email orders:** orders@ultimatedietsecrets.com
- **Postal orders:** Ultimate Diet Secrets, 68 Skyline Drive, Glen Mills, PA 19342
- **Website orders:** www.ultimatedietssecrets.com

Please send in your name and address if you want to be added to Dr. Ellis's mailing lists, either postal or email.

Name: _____

Address: _____

City: _____

State: _____ **Zip:** _____

Telephone: _____

Email address: _____

Payment: Check/MC/Visa/Amer. Express

Card number: _____

Name on card: _____

Expiration date: _____ / _____

Ultimate Diet Secrets.com
Dr. Gregory Ellis's 100% Weight Loss and Weight Control Solution

Quick Order Form

Fax Orders: 610-558-1287. Send this form.
Telephone Orders: Call 800-337-7041 (orders only). Have your credit card information ready.
email orders: orders@ultimatedietsecrets.com.
Postal orders: Ultimate Diet Secrets, 68 Skyline Drive, Glen Mills, PA 19342
Website orders: www.ultimatedietssecrets.com

Please send in your name and address if you want to be added to Dr. Ellis's mailing lists, either postal or email.

Name: _____

Address: _____

City: _____

State: _____ **Zip:** _____

Telephone: _____

Email address: _____

Payment: Check/MC/Visa/Amer. Express

Card number: _____

Name on card: _____

Expiration date: _____/_____